Purloined Organs

H. A. E. Zwart

Purloined Organs

Psychoanalysis of Transplant Organs as Objects of Desire

palgrave
macmillan

H. A. E. Zwart
Erasmus School of Philosophy
Erasmus University Rotterdam
Rotterdam, Zuid-Holland, The Netherlands

ISBN 978-3-030-05353-6   ISBN 978-3-030-05354-3   (eBook)
https://doi.org/10.1007/978-3-030-05354-3

Library of Congress Control Number: 2019934091

This Palgrave Pivot imprint is published by the registered company Springer Nature
Switzerland AG.
The registered company address is: Gewerbestrasse 11, 6330 Cham, Switzerland

CONTENTS

LIST OF FIGURES

CHAPTER 1

Introduction: Organ Recycling and Embodiment

Abstract Bioethical discourse on organ donation covers a wide range of topics, from informed consent procedures and scarcity issues up to transplant tourism and organ trade. Over the past decades, this discourse evolved into a stream of documents of immense proportions. Beneath the manifest level of discourse, a more latent dimension can be discerned, revolving around issues of embodiment, the status of the human body and the concept of bodily integrity. Here, the body emerges as something which we have, but at the same time are, and as something which constitutes a whole, while at the same time being a set of replaceable parts. This study examines transplantation discourse from an oblique perspective, using literature and cinema as high-resolution magnifying glasses.

Keywords Organ recycling • Embodiment • Bioethical • Depth ethics • Organ market • Oblique perspective

Bioethical discourse on organ donation and transplantation medicine covers a wide range of topics, from informed consent procedures and scarcity issues up to transplant tourism and organ trade. Over the past decades, this discourse evolved into a stream of documents of bewildering proportions, encompassing thousands of books, papers, conferences, blogs, consensus meetings, policy reports, media debates and other outlets. Beneath the manifest level of discourse, however, a more latent dimension can be

© The Author(s) 2019
H. A. E. Zwart, *Purloined Organs*,
https://doi.org/10.1007/978-3-030-05354-3_1

discerned, revolving around issues of embodiment, the moral status of the human body and the concept of bodily integrity. This publication aims to bring these "deeper" questions to the fore. What is envisioned is a "depth" ethics (the moral equivalent of a depth psychology) focussing on the tensions, conflicts and ambiguities at work in bioethical deliberations on organ transplantation, fuelling the viewpoints articulated on the more manifest levels of discourse. Organ donation reopens the question of the status of the body as something which we *have*, but at the same time *are*, and as something which constitutes a *whole*, while at the same time being a *set* of replaceable elements or parts.

Transplantation medicine affects the way in which we experience ourselves as embodied subjects (Blackman 2010; Shildrick 2010). Organ transplantation has "reconceptualised" (Scheper-Hughes 2000) our collective body image, notably by giving rise to a commodification of body parts, reframing the human body as a potential resource for organ recycling on behalf of suffering others and as a collection of separable, detachable, exchangeable and re-incorporable *partial objects* (Blackman 2010; Waldby and Mitchell 2006, p. 7; Rabinow 1996, p. 95). Seen through the eyes of transplantation medicine, the intimate interior of our bodies contains a set of valuable items which other humans (craving subjects) lack. And this tension between what potential donors *have* and what potential recipients desperately *need*, turns organs such as hearts and kidneys into valuable and procurable *objects of desire*. This is underscored by the fact that transplant organs (harvested either from living or from deceased donors) are currently available as merchandise on a clandestine but thriving global market: an international organ bazaar (Rheeder 2017). In his book *The Red Market*, Carney (2011) traces the contours of a multibillion-dollar global organ trafficking, although the actual extent of this world-spanning body shop remains an issue of dispute (Meyer 2006; Shimazono 2007; Scheper-Hughes 2008; Greenberg 2013).

Beyond the societal impact of transplantation medicine, often framed in bioethical terms, an ontological dimension can be discerned. Transplantation medicine reinforces (and at the same time builds on) a particular understanding of human embodiment, namely the view of the human body as an aggregate of replaceable, exchangeable and exploitable parts: items that should not be allowed to go waste. As Žižek (2004/2012) phrases it, due to the availability of heart, liver and other transplants, in combination with pacemakers, artificial limbs, transposable skin and similar items, a new type of body is emerging, a "body in pieces", a composite of replaceable components (p. 108). The plasticity of our body-image becomes more pronounced as human beings increasingly see themselves as "spare parts persons" (Schweda and Schicktanz 2009) whose bodies are collections of "detachable things" (Waldby 2002, p. 239). Seen from this perspective, organ trafficking (the emergence of a global clandestine organ market) is a symptom of a more comprehensive ontological event: the advent of the body as an organ recycling resource.

As Lesley Sharp (2006, 2007) has pointed out, transplantation medicine gives rise to two incommensurable discourses concerning the human body. On the one hand, it transforms procurable body parts into "objects of intense desire" (p. 49, p. 52). Human cadavers become lucrative treasure coves from which reusable parts can be harvested. A single body may contain fifty or more transplantable items. As transplant surgery is exorbitantly expensive, donated organs are objects of great value, bearing heavy price tags. And yet, both the surgical realities involved in removing organs from the torsos of donors and their economic costliness are obfuscated and mystified, Sharp argues, by euphemistic linguistic constructions— "semantic massage", as Richardson (1996) phrases it—which continue to revolve around vocabularies of "Samaritan" disinterested altruism and the "gift of life" (Hagen 1982). As a result, contemporary organ transplant discourse is permeated by a profound ontological tension: an "ideological disjunction" (Sharp 2006), between the commodifiable and the inviolable body, between lucrative and intrusive surgical practices on the one hand and a rhetoric of dignity and benevolence on the other.

To bring this ontological tension to the fore, a depth ethics is called for, bypassing (bracketing) the more immediate (manifest) ethical issues at hand, in order to focus on the more basic (latent) conceptual shifts that are unfolding on a different scene or stage—or "Schauplatz", to use the Freudian term (1900/1942, p. 541).[1] In order to open them up for critical reflection, I propose to examine transplantation discourse from an oblique perspective, using literature and cinema as high-resolution magnifying glasses (Zwart 2017). Movies and novels relate to contemporary culture in a way that is similar to how dreams or day-dreams relate to

---

[1] Whilst this study focusses on organ transplantation cinema as a "different scene", there are other alternative scenes where the uncanny dimensions of organ procurement are exposed. One unsettling example is China, where prisoners, notably followers of the spiritual Falun Gong movement, are systematically used as a human organ resource (Van Assche 2018; Matas and Trey 2012; Sharif et al. 2014), a practice which constitutes the reverse or perverse side of organ practices in the West (a sinister, etatist version of organ theft).

everyday consciousness, providing a stage where (evolving and conflict-
ing) understandings of human embodiment are enacted, probed and
questioned; provided that mechanisms such as condensation, displacement, representability and secondary elaboration (Freud 1900/1942) are
taken into account. These tensions and ambiguities will be addressed from
a psychoanalytical angle. Notably, the work of Jacques Lacan (1901–1981)
will be used to highlight some of the contradictions and ambivalences of
bodily existence surfacing in the contemporary transplantation debate.

The attempt to approach organ donation from a Lacanian perspective
may cause some raised eyebrows. To begin with, besides the interpretative
difficulties raised by the idiosyncrasy of his oeuvre, Lacan hardly ever
addressed topics such as organ donation or transplantation medicine, so
that the idea of extrapolating his views to such topics seems a hazardous
endeavour. Moreover, Lacan himself explicitly discards the feasibility of
"applied psychoanalysis", calling it a silly "deviation".[2] And yet, his work
teems with insights that may significantly enrich our understanding of the
various ambivalences entailed in the transplantation debate, so that it
would be an intellectual waste not to use his work as a resource (seeing it
solely as an object for academic "author studies"). Moreover, in one of his
Seminars, bearing the telling title *D'un Autre à l'autre* (from an Other to
the other), Lacan discusses organ harvesting quite explicitly (Lacan
1968–1969/2006). Given the fact, however, that bioethical quandaries
are seldomly addressed by him directly, a short introduction into his views
on embodiment will be an indispensable preparatory exercise. Subsequently,
I will elucidate these views with the help of bodily practices which are
more abundantly discussed in the psychoanalytical literature, and in
Lacan's writing in particular (and which, like organ donation, involve
"gifts of the body"), notably sexuality and Christianity. Building on this
conceptual framework, I will further develop my Lacanian approach to
transplantation medicine with the help of a series of case studies. Before
fleshing out my Lacanian viewpoint in more detail, however, I will first
outline the historical-ontological backdrop: the emergence (in philosophy,
literature and art) of the fractious body, whose integrity is both endangered and safeguarded by modern biomedicine.

---

[2] "Cette déviation bouffonne que j'espère barrer, qui est déjà étalée de longues années sous
le terme de psychanalyse appliquée" (1968–1969/2006, p. 66).

REFERENCES

Blackman, L. 2010. Bodily Integrity. *Body & Society* 16 (3): 1–9.

Carney, S. 2011. *The Red Market: On the Trail of the World's Organ Brokers, Bone Thieves, Blood Farmers, and Child Traffickers*. New York: HarperCollins.

Freud, S. 1900/1942. Die Traumdeutung. In *Gesammelte Werke II/III*. London: Imago.

Greenberg, O. 2013. The Global Organ Trade. *Cambridge Quarterly of Healthcare Ethics* 22 (3): 238–245.

Hagen, P.J. 1982. *Blood: Gift or Merchandise; Towards an International Blood Policy*. New York: Liss.

Lacan, J. 1968–1969/2006. *Le Séminaire de Jacques Lacan XVI: D'un Autre à l'autre*. Paris: Éditions du Seuil.

Matas, D., and T. Trey. 2012. *Transplant Abuse in China*. Niagara Falls: Seraphim Editions.

Meyer, S. 2006. Trafficking in Human Organs in Europe: A Myth or an Actual Threat? *European Journal of Crime, Criminal Law & Criminal Justice* 14 (2): 208–229.

Rabinow, P. 1996. *Essays on the Anthropology of Reason*. Princeton: Princeton University Press.

Rheeder, R. 2017. A Global Bioethical Perspective on Organ Trafficking: Discrimination, Stigmatisation and the Vulnerable. *South Africa Journal of Bioethics and Law* 10 (1): 20–24. https://doi.org/10.7196/SAJBL.2017. v10i1.528.

Richardson, R. 1996. Fearful Symmetry: Corpses for Anatomy, Organs for Transplantation? In *Organ Transplantation: Meanings and Realities*, ed. S. Youngner, R. Fox, and L. O'Connell, 66–100. Madison: University of Wisconsin Press.

Scheper-Hughes, N. 2000. The Global Traffic in Human Organs. *Current Anthropology* 41: 191–224.

———. 2008. *The Last Commodity: Post-Human Ethics, Global (In)Justice and the Traffic in Organs*. Penang: Multiversity & Citizens International.

Schweda, M., and S. Schicktanz. 2009. The 'Spare Parts Person'? Conceptions of the Human Body and Their Implications for Public Attitudes Towards Organ Donation and Organ Sale. *Philosophy, Ethics, and Humanities in Medicine* 4 (4): 1–10.

Sharif, A., M. Fiatarone Singh, T. Trey, and J. Lavee. 2014. Organ Procurement from Executed Prisoners in China. *American Journal of Transplantation* 14: 2246–2252.

Sharp, L. 2006. *Strange Harvest: Organ Transplants, Denatured Bodies and the Transformed Self*. Berkeley/Los Angeles/London: University of California Press.

————. 2007. *Bodies, Commodities and Biotechnologies. Death, Mourning and Scientific Desire in the Realm of Human Organ Transfer.* New York: Columbia University Press.

Shildrick, M. 2010. Some Reflections on the Socio-Cultural and Bioscientific Limits of Bodily Integrity. *Body & Society* 16 (3): 11–22.

Shimazono, Y. 2007. The State of the International Organ Trade: A Provisional Picture Based on Integration of Available Information. *Bulletin of the WHO* 85 (12). https://doi.org/10.1590/S0042-96862007001200017.

Van Assche, K. 2018. Combating the Trade in Organs: Why Should We Preserve the Communal Nature of Organ Transplantation. In *Personalized Medicine, Individual Choice and the Common Good*, ed. B. van Beers, D. Dickenson, and S. Sterckx, 77–112. Cambridge: Cambridge University Press.

Waldby, C. 2002. Biomedicine, Tissue Transfer and Intercorporeality. *Feminist Theory* 3: 235–250.

Waldby, C., and R. Mitchell. 2006. *Tissue Economies: Blood, Organs and Cell Lines in Late Capitalism.* Durham & London: Duke University Press.

Žižek, S. 2004/2012. *Organs Without Bodies: On Deleuze and Consequences.* London/New York: Routledge.

Zwart, H. 2017. The Oblique Perspective: Philosophical Diagnostics of Contemporary Life Sciences Research. *Life Sciences, Society & Policy* 13 (1): 1–20. https://doi.org/10.1186/s40504-017-0047-9.

CHAPTER 2

The Body As an Aggregate of Replaceable Parts

Abstract Western understandings of human embodiment are adrift. The traditional (Christian) view, emphasising the integrity (wholeness, inviolability) of the human body, is challenged by the ontology of contemporary techno-science, exemplified by transplantation medicine.

The emergence of the body as an aggregate of parts is both prepared and questioned by genres of the imagination, notably literary documents such as *The dream of d'Alembert*, written by Denis Diderot in 1769, and *Frankenstein*, published by Mary Wollstonecraft Shelley in 1818. Since then, transplantation medicine has evolved from utopia (or dystopia) into science.

Keywords Body as aggregate • Inviolable body • Body ontology • Christianity • Organ shortage • Blood transfusion

Current Western understandings of human embodiment are adrift. The traditional (Christian) view, emphasising the integrity (wholeness, inviolability) of the human body, is challenged by (the implicit ontology of) contemporary techno-science, exemplified by transplantation medicine (Zwart 2000, 2014, 2016). In this chapter, the history of this dramatic ontological transition will be outlined.

To come to terms with the unsettling vulnerability (corruptibility) of the *real* human body, Christianity developed the idea of an inviolable *ideal* body, salvageable and restorable through divine intervention (Zwart 2000). Saint Paul explains (1 Corinthians 12:12–20) that, although the body has many parts, they remain firmly embedded within the body as a whole. They cannot step out and detach themselves from their corporeal embeddedness. It is not possible for a foot or an ear (as *partial objects*) to say, "I do not belong to this body", Paul argues. They cannot stop being part of the body as such. In short: many parts, one body. And this has normative implications as well, for Christians are summoned to safeguard the wholeness of their own bodies as well as those of others, as a preparatory exercise for the eventual transfiguration (sublation or sublimation) of the real (corruptible) body into an unperishable new version, on Resurrection Day, as envisioned by Christianity. In the context of mundane existence, however, bodily integrity can already be fostered through ascetic exercises and self-care, living up to the ideal. As Michel Foucault (1994) phrased it, during the Christian era the "manly" (ancient Greek and Roman) model of body-management as a form of self-mastery gave way to a more "feminine" model, emphasising the preservation of intactness (of the unviolated, literally "untouched" body).

This may seem at odds with juxtaposed features of Christianity such as the willingness of Christ to accept corporeal violations brought about by crucifixion or of Christian martyrs to endure corporeal torture, depriving them of their breasts (Saint Agatha), eyes (Saint Lucia), skin (Saint Bartholomew) or other body parts. But again, such impairments (brought about by a godless cultural environment) merely affected the real and vulnerable body, not the transfigured one, which will be bestowed on believers by way of restitution during resurrection: a leap-like transfiguration which will take no more than an "atom" of time (1 Kor. 14–15).

In modern times, this ancient idea of bodily integrity was drastically reframed by biomedicine, notably by immunology research. In immunological discourse, "integrity" no longer refers to the image of the body as an inviolable whole, but rather to the real and active (observable, molecular and quantifiable) processes that protect us from external intrusions, via organismal surveillance: the immune system, represented by the lymphocytes first and foremost, through which the "integrity" of the organism is actively maintained (Burnet 1963, p. vi). Nonetheless, human beings can still foster corporeal integrity through self-care (personal hygiene and lifestyle, for instance). Paradoxically, however, by revealing the biomolecular mechanisms of integrity maintenance, immunology at the same time undermines bodily integrity, for example, by developing methods to bypass or repress immune responses (to forgo rejection of implanted organs). Thus, in the end, biomedicine has propagated the understanding of the human body as an aggregate of removable (replaceable) parts, rather than as an integer (inviolable, impenetrable) whole.

The emergence of this (now dominant) view is also reflected, endorsed and questioned by genres of the imagination, notably literary documents, preparing the ground for the birth of modern biomedicine, such as *Le Rêve de d'Alembert* ("The dream of d'Alembert"), written by Denis Diderot in 1769 anticipating key biomedical developments (Diderot 1769/1951), but also *Frankenstein; or, the Modern Prometheus*, published by Mary Wollstonecraft Shelley in 1818 (1818/1968). Although both works are quite different in terms of mood and style—in the sense that, whereas Diderot's oneiric delirium heralds the emerging life sciences with enthusiasm, Frankenstein's elaborate confession rather invokes anxiety and unease—they convey a similar, anticipatory message. In both documents, one and the same basic view of embodiment is brought to the fore: the (human) body is *not* an indivisible unity, but rather an aggregate of replaceable parts. Indeed, one could argue that, ever since, biomedical life sciences are dedicated to verify the basic validity of this ontological claim. Resistance against this (inevitable) transition stems from the fact that it actually represents an ontological trauma: a narcissistic offence which undermines the image of the body as an uncompromised whole, paving the way towards fragmentation and disintegration.

Organ transplantation has played a prominent role in the unfolding of this narrative, with blood donation as an opening chapter. During the (Victorian) nineteenth century, experiments with blood transfusion (as an alternative to blood-letting: as blood-letting in reverse) often gave rise to disastrous results, as is reflected in Bram Stoker's novel *Dracula*, published in 1895: a story about a young gentleman-physician who donates blood (as a substitute/displacement for semen, perhaps) to his ailing fiancée (Lucy Westenra, the recipient). Before the intervention, the latter displays symptoms strikingly similar to the ones portrayed as "hysteria" by Breuer and Freud in the same period (Freud 1895/1952). In Stoker's novel, however, Lucy's unsettling condition quickly deteriorates, but her status as a semi-comatose "undead" is not attributed to blood poisoning, but to an uncanny, demonic, inexorable force named vampirism (Zwart 2018). When in the year 1900 Karl Landsteiner discovers blood types, this not only makes blood transfusion safer, but also effectively transfers vampirism from the Victorian boudoir to the realm of horror cinema. At the same time, it unleashes an insatiable desire for human blood, a growing medical demand, which has never subsided ever since. Indeed, one could argue that, building on Landsteiner's discovery, modern biomedicine itself became an institutionalised mega-vampire, displaying an excessive techno-scientific craving for human blood.

This is fleshed out in the science fiction novel *The Red Star* by Russian communist Alexander Bogdanov (1908/1984), who used blood transfusion as a core ingredient of his utopian society, situated on Mars, the Red Planet, functioning as an imaginative laboratory to explore the *red* (i.e. communist) future (Groys and Hagemeister 2005). Whereas Earthlings perform blood donations merely for "philanthropic" reasons (Bogdanov (1908/1984, p. 86)), procuring blood from the healthy in order to save the lives of the ill, Bogdanov's Martians routinely perform mutual blood transfusions between healthy individuals, pumping blood from one person into another and back again, as a means of rejuvenation, to increase productivity and life expectancy—eventually fusing human bodies into one gigantic super-organism, one collectivised workforce. Bogdanov himself died in 1928, after a foundering blood transfusion experiment.

Other important landmark events in the process of opening up the human body as an aggregate of procurable and reusable parts were the first kidney transplants (in the 1950s), the first heart and liver transplants (in the 1960s), the introduction of the brain-death concept (in 1968, prompted by the surgical desire to facilitate organ procurement) and the discovery of cyclosporine (in 1972). Step by step, the dream of the reusable body began to move from dream to reality and from utopia to science (Zwart 2009). As Margaret Lock (2002) convincingly argued, transplantation medicine involves a dramatic shift of attention from the body of the (brain-dead) donor to the latter's living, detachable, procurable *organs*. Care for the organs, rather than for the (violated) body becomes the dominant concern. In stark contrast to the pale and life-less exterior of the brain-dead donor, the latter's disclosed interior remains colourful, warm and alive during the operation, and the transplant team emphatically focuses its attention on the alluring, healthy organs, ready to be harvested (p. 21), too valuable to be used for just one life alone (p. 81). By removing them from the body, they become decontextualised and commoditised. Already in 1967, it was predicted that organ shortage would become the biggest challenge of transplantation medicine. Lock cites a *New York Times* article commenting on the first heart transplant: "One need not be a science fiction writer to envision the possibility of future murder rings supplying healthy organs for black-market surgeons whose patients are unwilling to wait until natural sources have supplied the heart or liver or pancreas they need" (2002, p. 83). Indeed, humans were becoming "puzzle people", as pioneer transplantation surgeon Thomas Starzl (1992/2003) phrased it: potential multiple organ donors and/or recipients.

This stepwise biomedical disruption/subversion of the traditional understanding of the human body as an integer whole has strengthened the view of the body as an aggregate of replaceable parts (the inherent metaphysics of transplantation medicine), resulting in a commodification of the body and allowing individuals to see organs and tissues (of themselves and of others) as valuable resources, even as things for sale. This especially pertains to surplus parts: organs, tissues and other bodily items which living humans (in principle) can do without. Resistance against commodification of body parts is often grounded in ontological convictions which stress the dignity and integrity (wholeness, inviolability) of the body as such: the Christian view in short, albeit often clad in secularised wordings, so that the ontological battle (the gigantomachia) between old and new visions of embodiment is still ongoing. As Žižek (2004/2012) phrases it, even if we try to keep our distance to the "black hole" that is opened up by biomedical science, subverting our most basic moral notions, the fact that the human body has been "deprived of its former impenetrable density" cannot be undone (p. 111). Therefore, he argues, rather than clinging to traditional convictions, it seems preferable to "tarry with the negative" and to explore what practices of embodiment are currently emerging.

References

Bogdanov, A. 1908/1984. *Red Star.* Bloomington: University of Indiana Press.

Burnet, F.M. 1963. *The Integrity of the Body.* Cambridge: Harvard University Press.

Diderot, D. 1769/1951. *Le rêve de d'Alembert: entretien entre d'Alembert et Diderot.* Société des textes français modernes. Paris: Didier.

Foucault, M. 1994. A propos de la généalogie de l'éthique. In *Dits et Écrits IV*, 383–411. Paris: Gallimard.

Freud, S. 1895/1952. Studien über Hysterie. In *Gesammelte Werke I*, 75–312. London: Imago.

Groys, B., and M. Hagemeister. 2005. *Die neue Menschheit: Biopolitische Utopien in Russland zu Beginn des 20.* Jahrhunderts. Frankfurt am Main: Suhrkamp.

Lock, M. 2002. *Twice Dead: Organ Transplants and the Reinvention of Death.* Berkeley/Los Angeles/California: University of California Press.

Starzl, T. 1992/2003. *The Puzzle People. Memoirs of a Transplant Surgeon.* Pittsburgh/London: University of Pittsburgh Press.

Žižek, S. 2004/2012. *Organs Without Bodies: On Deleuze and Consequences.* London/New York: Routledge.

Zwart, H. 2000. From Circle to Square: Integrity, Vulnerability and Digitalization. In *Bioethics and Law II: Four Ethical Principles*, ed. P. Kemp et al., 141–153. Copenhagen: Rhodos.

———. 2009. From Utopia to Science: Challenges of Personalised Genomics Information for Health Management and Health Enhancement. *Medicine Studies* 1 (2): 155–166.

———. 2014. The Donor Organ as an 'Object A': A Lacanian Perspective on Organ Donation and Transplantation Medicine. *Medicine, Health Care & Philosophy: A European Journal* 17 (4): 559–571. https://doi.org/10.1007/s11019-014-9553-1.

———. 2016. Transplantation Medicine, Organ Theft Cinema and Bodily Integrity. *Subjectivity* 9 (2): 151–180. https://doi.org/10.1057/sub.2016.1.

———. 2018. Vampires, Viruses and Verbalisation: Bram Stoker's Dracula as a Genealogical Window into Fin-De-Siècle Science. *Janus Head: Journal of Interdisciplinary Studies in Literature, Continental Philosophy, Phenomenological Psychology, and the Arts* 16 (2): 14–53.

CHAPTER 3

An Ontological Struggle: Integrity Versus Fragmentation

Abstract Building on the previous chapter, this chapter traces the emergence of the body as a collection or aggregate of replaceable and procurable parts. Special attention will be given to Scholastic and modern understandings of embodiment, fleshed out by Aquinas and Kant, but also to a famous portrayal of human embodiment by painter Jeroen Bosch. This allows us to fathom how this ontological transition has turned organs (such as hearts and kidneys) into valuable and procurable objects of desire, introducing a tension between what potential donors have and what potential recipients desperately need. This is underscored by the fact that transplant organs (harvested either from living or from deceased donors) are currently available as merchandise on a global organ market.

Keywords Bodily integrity • Thomas Aquinas • Hieronymus Bosch
• Garden of Eden • Garden of Earthly Delights • Immanuel Kant
• Self-mutilation • Partial suicide

During the 1950s and 1960s, when the first kidney, heart and liver transplants were conducted, Neo-Scholastic views of embodiment were still quite influential in occidental debates, although their discursive sway soon began to wane. Building on Thomas Aquinas and others, the body was conceived in terms of integrity and wholeness, and commodification was out of the question. Human individuals were seen as stewards rather than

© The Author(s) 2019
H. A. E. Zwart, *Purloined Organs*,
https://doi.org/10.1007/978-3-030-05354-3_3

owners of their bodies and expected to manage their body in such a manner that its inherent intactness was respected (Zwart 2000, 2016).

Yet, contrary to still widely accepted views (which associate experimentation with modernity), the late-medieval (gothic) period already combined conceptual scholarship (i.e. scholasticism) with experimental work. The experimental method (*scientia experimentalis*) already flourished in late-medieval monastic settings, represented by medieval scholars such as Albert the Great, Roger Bacon, Duns Scotus and Cusanus (Grant 1974), who already endorsed mechanistic perspectives on embodiment. In fact, Thomas himself already compares living beings to clockworks (*horologia*) and machines (Zwart 1997, p. 381). Thus, late-medieval ontology was already challenged by the tension between the inviolable body (the traditional Christian view) and its emerging counterpart, bent on exploration and fragmentation of the body.

This is reflected by a well-known art-work, the famous triptych known as *The Garden of Earthly Delights* by Hieronymus Bosch, painted somewhere between 1490 and 1510 (Zwart 2016). This imaginative collage of colourful scenes, projected on a triple screen, could be considered a late-medieval "movie": an artistic, quasi-cinematic enactment of the ontological struggle over embodiment. While the left panel depicts Adam and Eve *in statu innocentiae*, as Aquinas phrased it (1922, Pars Ia, Q 96–97), the right panel (with its horrible scenes of warfare, torture and prostitution) envisions the catastrophe awaiting us when bodies are regarded as something that can be exploited, mutilated and spoiled at will. The central (transitional) panel seems especially relevant for our purposes. Here, the integrity of (naked) human bodies is endangered by various earthly temptations.

One of these temptations is the *cupido sciendi*, that is, the will to know—more concretely, the urge to acquire insight into the body by conducting experiments. There are various experiments depicted on this panel, besides erotic ones, including an animal experiment involving a test tube and a rat, but multiple experiments can be detected once we begin to look for them. Various pieces of laboratory equipment, such as glass tubes and distillation vessels, can be discerned (Dixon 1981): a foreboding of the imminent subversion of bodily integrity through experimentation. The body has lost its innocence and the famous triptych enacts the ontological collision between traditional (scriptural) and experimental (in vitro) understandings of embodiment. A three-act drama can be discerned, from integrity (left panel), via experiments, erotic dreams and worldly temptations (the central panel) down to the disconcerting prospect of the dismantled body, exposed to dismemberment and fragmentation (right panel).

During the Enlightenment era, the issue of bodily integrity was taken up by Immanuel Kant, among others. Although he presents human agents in an almost disembodied manner, as bodies without organs as it were, Kant (1785/1980) does pay attention to bodily integrity, and even discusses the commodification of body parts, using teeth and hair as key examples, seeing the selling/buying of the latter as slightly less objectionable than the former. In the light of human dignity, Kant argues, body parts are not for sale. Bodily integrity limits the modern tendency to transform all objects into commodities. Body parts are priceless; their value cannot be captured in market terms. Kant also discusses self-mutilation, notably self-castration by male sopranos. According to Kant, we are not entitled to disrupt the body's wholeness for short-term gain, since self-mutilation is self-contradictory: it is a use of freedom which undermines the physical conditions of freedom and autonomy. Indeed, he considers self-mutilation (for profit; an exemption is made for medical considerations) as *partial suicide* (1785/1980, p. 555), discarding it as wholly unjustifiable, because it actually undermines human agency. For Kant, the removal/selling of spare/surplus body parts is at odds with (our obligation to respect) human dignity in our own person.

There are risks involved, however. As Lacan (1966, p. 765 ff., 1959–1960/1986) has argued, a basic congruence may be discerned between Immanuel Kant and Marquis de Sade. In the latter's oeuvre, the maxim that one may (or indeed *should*) exploit (the bodies of) others for the maximisation of universal pleasure is framed as a categorical imperative, while resistance against the consistency of such as scheme is discarded as "pathological" (i.e. irrational) sentimentalism. For Kant, however, such a sadistic turn is sufficiently contained by the obligation to respect humanity in one's own person and that of others. This should ward off the prospect of a sadistic universe (i.e. the sardonic right panel of *The Garden of Earthly Delights*). But whereas Kant's ontology still seems to adhere to traditional convictions concerning the dignity and integrity of the human body as a whole, under the sway of biomedicine the vicissitudes of human embodiment are bound to move in a juxtaposed direction. As Jacques-Alain Miller (2001) phrases it, transplantation surgery is fundamentally at odds with our desire to celebrate the unity of the body. What is actually in progress is the contrary: the cutting up and dismemberment of the body through medical power, the emergence of the "body in pieces". Indeed, an ontological landscape is currently unfolding in which the understanding of organs as commodities has become much more plausible than Kant was willing to acknowledge. Let this suffice as a short genealogical account of the ontological shift from the body as an integer whole to the body as a collection of removable parts. In the next chapters, Lacan's psychoanalytic understanding of human embodiment will be fleshed out.

REFERENCES

Aquinas, T. 1922. *Summa Theologica*. Taurini: Marietti.

Dixon, L. 1981. Bosch's Garden of Delights Triptych: Remnants of a Fossil Science. *The Art Bulletin* 63 (1): 96–113.

Grant, E. 1974. *A Source Book in Medieval Science*. Harvard: Harvard University Press.

Kant, I. 1785/1980. Grundlegung zur Metaphysik der Sitten. In *Werkausgabe 7*. Frankfurt am Main: Suhrkamp.

Lacan, J. 1959–1960/1986. *Le Séminaire de Jacques Lacan VII: L'éthique de la psychanalyse*. Paris: Éditions du Seuil.

———. 1966. Kant avec Sade. In *Écrits*, 765–790. Paris: Éditions du Seuil.

Miller, J.-A. 2001. Lacanian Biology and the Event of the Body. *Lacanian Ink* 18: 6–29.

Zwart, H. 1997. What Is an Animal? A Philosophical Reflection on the Possibility of a Moral Relationship with Animals. *Environmental Values* 6 (4): 377–392.

———. 2000. From Circle to Square: Integrity, Vulnerability and Digitalization. In *Bioethics and Law II: Four Ethical Principles*, ed. P. Kemp et al., 141–153. Copenhagen: Rhodos.

———. 2016. Transplantation Medicine, Organ Theft Cinema and Bodily Integrity. *Subjectivity* 9 (2): 151–180. https://doi.org/10.1057/sub.2016.1.

CHAPTER 4

The Real, the Imaginary and the Symbolic: Lacan's Understanding of Embodiment

Abstract In this chapter, the ambiguities and tensions of human embodiment will be addressed from a psychoanalytical perspective, notably building on the work of Jacques Lacan, who distinguishes three realms or registers of bodily experience, three basic ways in which the human body comes to the fore and may be encountered in various practices, namely the *real* body, the *imaginary* body and the *symbolic* body. The *real* body is basically a fragmented body: a composite aggregate of organs, fluids, processes and products. The *imaginary* body refers to the body as a meaningful, aestheticised whole. Finally, the *symbolic* body is the body as it emerges in modern scientific research practices, measured, qualified and quantified with the help of biomedical equipment.

Keywords Lacanian psychoanalysis • Jacques Lacan • The imaginary • The symbolic • The real • Fragmented body • Mirror experience • Vesalius • Karl Landsteiner • Blood types • Symbolisation of the body • Partial objects

Lacan (1966) distinguishes three realms (or registers) of bodily experience, three basic ways in which the human body comes to the fore and may be encountered in various practices, namely the *real* body, the *imaginary* body and the *symbolic* body (Zwart 1998). The *real* body is basically experienced as a fragmented body: a composite aggregate of organs, fluids,

© The Author(s) 2019
H. A. E. Zwart, *Purloined Organs*,
https://doi.org/10.1007/978-3-030-05354-3_4

processes and products. The *imaginary* body, by contrast, refers to the body as a meaningful, aestheticised whole. Now, the body is envisioned in terms of integrity or wholeness and seen as an integrated unity. Finally, the *symbolic* body is the body as it emerges in modern scientific research practices, the body that is disclosed by technology and science, that is measured, qualified and quantified with the help of biomedical equipment. I will now explore these three registers/dimensions of human bodily experience somewhat further, with the help of some examples.

In everyday adult life, we are hardly ever directly confronted with the real, fragmented body. Rather, the fragmented body (corps morcelée) is the body as it is experienced by very young children during early stages of development, although it continues to emerge in the folds and margins of bodily experiences later in life.[1] The real body is that which resists efforts towards idealisation of the human body (scientific, artistic, religious or otherwise): it is unclean rather than clean, damaged rather than unviolated, destitute rather than wholesome, eerie rather than familiar.

A first effort to turn the fragmented body into a stable, coherent unity or whole is thematised by Lacan as the mirror experience (Lacan 1966, p. 93 ff.). By recognising their image in a mirror, Lacan argues, very young children for the first time learn to see themselves as complete individuals. This triumph over fragmentation gives rise to an experience of "jubilation". Yet, this newly acquired sense of unity is dependent on an external image, the *Gestalt* or *image* reflected in a mirror, and therefore remains highly vulnerable and image-dependent (imaginary).

The imaginary body can also be encountered in works of art, such as ancient Greek and Roman sculptures (or their Baroque or Neo-Classicist equivalents). An artistic rendering of the human body may present it as an integrated unity, as something admirable, stable and whole. Moreover, through various body practices, such as body-building, for example, athletes (male or female) may sculpt their bodies into living works of art, thus mimicking or mirroring examples (either in marble or in the flesh) presented by others. Ancient Greek statues were basically the statues of athletes or of gods (which amounted to the same thing, since gods were regarded as athletes and athletes as gods). Moreover, as Lacan explains, statues of human beings, erected alongside major roads in ancient times,

---

[1] This was already pointed out by Freud: "Die Pathologie lehrt uns [Fälle] kennen, in denen uns Teile des eigenen Körpers ... wie fremd und dem Ich nicht zugehörig erscheinen" (1930/1948, pp. 423–424).

conveyed a normative ideal, presenting integrity and dignity as basic normative attributes (Lacan 1955–1956/1981, p. 328; Cf. Zwart 2000). Thus, statues of heroes, emperors and other exemplary humans (both physically and morally) spread the ancient gospel of human dignity, of *humanitas*. They incorporated an idealised view of what embodied human beings should aspire to become. These statues were erected alongside public roads by way of ethical propaganda. They functioned like missionaries in stone, whose silent sermons made a definite impact on anonymous masses of travellers and passers-by (Cf. Sloterdijk 2009, p. 37 ff.). The idea of human dignity (as well as the commandment to respect and admire it) was thus carved into stone. In psychoanalytical language, human physical perfection was a result of artistic sublimation, turning flesh into marble. It was the celebration of the imaginary body: of a particular (normative) image of what our bodies ideally should look like. Turn thyself into a work of art! Ancient statues propagated a basic *idea* of what human bodies essentially *are*. Michelangelo's *David*, but also his impressive sculpture *Night* (in the *Sagrestia nuova* in Florence) may stand out as early modern counterparts (Cf. Cassell 1992).

The beautified body was not only celebrated by pagan (Greco-Roman) artistic representations and their modern equivalents, but also by Christian views of embodiment, although here a dramatic historical dimension was added. According to Thomas Aquinas for instance, the human body was once (*in statu innocentiae*, i.e. in Paradise) beautiful and whole, but we damaged and corrupted this beautiful work of art, this gift from God (1922, Pars Ia, Q 96–97). And now, it is our duty to restore our body to its state of original splendour, although this calls for divine support, a combination of human virtue and heavenly grace. Meanwhile, our earthly frame remains constantly under siege, exposed to corruptive forces, so that its fragile, vulnerable wholeness can never be taken for granted. Bodily existence entails a continuous struggle between good and evil, beauty and obscenity, consolidation and fragmentation.

The body as a *fragmented* body is played out in a highly provocative manner in Mary Wollstonecraft Shelley's novel *Frankenstein*, mentioned earlier and published precisely two centuries ago in 1818 (not coincidentally during the gestation period of modern medicine). A science student named Victor Frankenstein (whose mother died during delivery) decides to find out whether deceased human bodies can be brought to life again with the help of experimental science. We see him roaming cemeteries and mortuaries at night, looking for suitable bodily parts, organs and tissues.

From these collected parts, an organic amalgam is composed. Subsequently, by exposing it to high voltage electricity, this aggregate of organs is revivified, and the famous Monster is created, whose distorted torso suddenly starts to breathe and move. In other words, in Mary Shelley's novel, the body emerges as an *aggregate of replaceable parts*. This break-down of the unified, integer body into detachable, semi-autonomous bodily parts arouses a particular experience, which Freud refers to as "the uncanny" (1919/1947): a typical ingredient of horror stories. What Saint Paul considered impossible, is suddenly made possible: body parts may suddenly detach themselves from their corporeal embeddedness, presenting themselves as separate entities.

The ground for this experience of fractious embodiment had been prepared by early modern anatomists, by pioneers such as Vesalius (van den Berg 1961; Zwart 2002). Through dissection, the human body was opened up, so that the various parts and organs were exposed and presented as more or less separate entities (organs without a subject). And indeed, in plastic anatomical models produced for educational purposes, heart, lungs, liver, kidneys and other organs can easily be removed: they can be taken out, and subsequently placed back again. The organs involved are allowed to stand out, as it were: they have become distinguishable, in principle, from the body as a whole. Whereas modern anatomy disassembles the body into constituent parts, Victor Frankenstein rather worked the other way around: his aim was to reassemble a body from dispersed fragments.

Modern science opened up a new and unprecedented experience of bodily existence—distancing itself both from the chaotic and uncontrollable *real* body (experienced in early childhood and projected onto a distant, mythological past) and from the idealised and beautified *imaginary* body (reflected in the mirror experience, but also in classical sculpture as we have seen)—namely the *symbolic* body, describable with the help of mathematical, physiological and biochemical symbols. Now, the human body is measured, for instance, in terms of height and weight.[2] Gradually, notably in the nineteenth and twentieth centuries, a plethora of

---

[2] This register of bodily experience was opened up by Sanctorius (1561–1636), founding father of iatrophysics, whose notes on medical statics—*De Medicina Statica Aphorismis*—were published in 1614, after having spent 30 years of his life in a weighing chair, carefully measuring the effects of food intake and other daily habits on body weight, comparing it with the weight of waste products such as urine and faeces (Van den Berg 1961; Zwart 2016).

measurement practices emerged, establishing normal standard values for various bodily functions, such as oxygen saturation in the blood or systolic and diastolic blood pressure (120/80 mmHg). Outcomes of such measurements are represented with the help of specific symbols (kg, lbs, metre, cm, mmHg, etc.). Speaking about blood, an important step towards blood transfusion (as a preliminary form of transplantation medicine) was already discussed earlier, namely the discovery of blood types by Karl Landsteiner in 1900, describing blood samples in terms of the presence or absence of antigenic substances on the surface of red blood cells, represented by a minimal alphabet of symbols (A, B, AB and O). These myriads of symbols and measurements can be employed in mathematical equations, presenting one series of measurements as a function of another—for instance using weight and height to determine the body-mass index (BMI), as a way of describing, in short-hand, the basic condition of a particular human body. All these numbers, units, symbols, technical terms and acronyms constitute a symbolic ambiance, a symbolic environment referred to by Lacan as the *symbolic order*. It fosters particular ways of presenting the body, allowing it to emerge in a certain manner. Various technical instruments have been designed, ranging from standard medical equipment to fairly advanced high-tech devices and self-tracking gadgets, to support this ongoing symbolisation of the body in the context of biomedical science. This is what critics of contemporary techno-medicine are pointing to when they claim, for instance, that biomedical technologies endanger the dignity and integrity of the human body. The imaginary body (the body as a meaningful unity or whole) is disrupted by these powerful symbolic representations of the body, opening it up to calculated interventions and effective manipulations.

This not only affects the way we actually see and experience our bodies but entails far-reaching normative implications as well. Whereas a traditional (Greco-Roman or Christian) ontological evaluation of the body will emphasise unity, wholeness and integrity, the sway of modern science inevitably disperses the body into fragments. Organs emerge as *partial objects* (as Lacan, building on other authors such as Freud, Abraham and Klein, phrases it)—items detachable from the body as a *Gesamtbild*, that is, as a coherent, integrated whole. It is the return of the Frankensteinian vision of the body, but now under highly advanced techno-scientific conditions. Indeed, in this new scientific version, the fragmented body is no longer experienced as chaotic, incontrollable and unclean. Quite the contrary, it is meticulously described, analysed and sterilised, cleansed and purified by techno-science. Due to the dominance of the symbolic body, the real body fades into the backdrop (without ever being abolished completely).

One of the most symptomatic implications of this transition from the *real* and the *imaginary* to the *symbolic* body are contemporary discussions concerning ownership of the body and its multiple fragments. Whereas we can no longer claim ownership over a human body as a whole (as in the case of slavery), the ownership of bodily parts and fragments (of *partial organs*) increasingly became a matter of dispute (ten Have and Welie 1998). A world-famous, highly symptomatic example is of course the dispute over the ownership of the so-called HeLa cell lines (Skloot 2011; Horbach and Halffman 2017). There is evidently something uncanny in the idea that human cells or tissues can be cultivated and immortalised, analysed and owned in a laboratory environment while the person from whose body these cells were originally procured (Henrietta Lacks) died more than 60 years ago (in 1951). Besides the biomedical institutes that cure them, care for them and study them, individuals themselves may also claim ownership over bodily parts (tissues, fluids, DNA, extirpated organs, etc.), for instance in the context of biomedical research (Dekkers and ten Have 1998). Thus, the symbolisation of the body on the epistemological level inevitably calls for a concurrent symbolisation of the body on the ethical and legal level as well, in the form of laws, regulations, stipulations, ownership contracts, transfer agreements, informed consent procedures and so on. Not only must the physiological, endocrinological, anatomical and genetic features of bodily existence be minutely described, but its legal parameters must also be documented and ascertained as meticulously as possible.

REFERENCES

Aquinas, T. 1922. *Summa Theologica*. Taurini: Marietti.

van den Berg, J.H. 1961. *Het menselijk lichaam: een metabletisch onderzoek 2: Het verlaten lichaam*. Nijkerk: Callenbach.

Cassell, E. 1992. The Body of the Future. In *The Body in Medical Thought and Practice*, Philosophy & Medicine, ed. D. Leder, vol. 43, 233–249. Dordrecht/Boston/London: Kluwer.

Dekkers, W., and H. ten Have. 1998. Biomedical Research with Human Body 'Parts'. In *Ownership of the Human Body: Philosophical Considerations of the Human Body and Its Parts in Healthcare*, ed. H. ten Have and J. Welie, 49–63. Dordrecht/Boston/London: Kluwer.

Freud, S. 1919/1947. Das Unheimliche. In *Gesammelte Werke XII*, 227–268. London: Imago.

———. 1930/1948. Das Unbehagen in der Kultur. In *Gesammelte Werke XIV*, 419–513. London: Imago.

Horbach, S., and W. Halffman. 2017. The Ghosts of HeLa: How Cell Line Misidentification Contaminates the Scientific Literature. *PLoS One* 12 (10): e0186281. https://doi.org/10.1371/journal.pone.0186281.

Lacan, J. 1955–1956/1981. *Le Séminaire de Jacques Lacan III: Les psychoses.* Paris: Éditions du Seuil.

———. 1966. *Écrits.* Paris: Éditions du Seuil.

Skloot, R. 2011. *The Immortal Life of Henrietta Lacks.* New York: Broadway Paperbacks.

Sloterdijk, P. 2009. *Du musst dein Leben ändern: Über Anthropotechnik.* Frankfurt: Suhrkamp.

Ten Have, H., and J. Welie. 1998. *Ownership of the Human Body: Philosophical Considerations of the Human Body and Its Parts in Healthcare.* Dordrecht/Boston/London: Kluwer.

Zwart, H. 1998. Medicine, Symbolization and the 'Real Body': Lacan's Understanding of Medical Science. *Medicine, Healthcare and Philosophy: A European Journal* 1 (2): 107–117.

———. 2000. From Circle to Square: Integrity, Vulnerability and Digitalization. In *Bioethics and Law II: Four Ethical Principles*, ed. P. Kemp et al., 141–153. Copenhagen: Rhodos.

———. 2002. *Boude bewoordingen. De historische fenomenologie van J.H. van den Berg.* Kampen: Klement/Kapellen: Pelckmans. ISBN 90 77070 26 5.

———. 2016. The Obliteration of Life: Depersonalisation and Disembodiment in the Terabyte Age. *New Genetics and Society* 35 (1): 69–89. https://doi.org/1 0.1080/14636778.2016.1143770.

CHAPTER 5

Love and the Idealisation of the Body

Abstract Before focussing on transplantation medicine as such, we will consider bodily practices which have been discussed more extensively by psychoanalysis, first of all eroticism and love, which involve an idealisation or sublimation of the body, but may also a focus on (or be even obsessed with) specific body parts as partial objects. If such objects come too close, however, as stand-alone entities, separated from the body as a whole, these objects of desire become uncanny.

Keywords Idealisation • Partial objects • Objects of desire • Matheme of desire • The uncanny

In terms of body practices, while organ transplantation is hardly discussed in psychoanalysis, there has always been an emphasis on sexuality and love. Before turning to organ donation proper therefore, the role of the body in sexuality will be given due attention. To begin with, Lacan emphasises that love and eroticism often involve overestimation, investing the body of the beloved Other with surplus value, transforming it into a unique, sublime, almost supernatural *imaginary* body. This idealised and elevated body plays a prominent role in sexual relationships. Lacan even goes so far as to claim that a sexual relationship (between lover and beloved) is strictly speaking impossible because of its dependence on the imaginary body. In the case of narcissism (the love of self), a substantial amount of libido is

© The Author(s) 2019
H. A. E. Zwart, *Purloined Organs,*
https://doi.org/10.1007/978-3-030-05354-3_5

invested in one's own body, so that the bodily self becomes the object of love, care and desire, turning it into a living work of art, through diet, lifestyle, exercises and so on. Satisfaction may be derived from touching and caressing one's own body, or from viewing its reflection in a mirror. To the extent that others are involved, these others may become a second self: an exemplification of what we ourselves aspire to be, the (in vivo) paragon of our (unconscious) ideal of human embodiment in its most impeccable state. Thus, narcissism is closely connected with erotic devotion: it is a celebration of the imaginary body as a perfect *Gesamtbild*.

We may also see the beloved other really as *other*, however, that is: as significantly different from ourselves. Such an Other seems to provide us with the very thing we lack or seek. For instance, someone whose bodily and mental features compensate our own inferiorities, our weaknesses and flaws. The Other (the erotic object) now emerges as our complement. We experience our body not in terms of wholeness (A), but rather in terms of deprivation ($Å$). We are yearning for a desirable but indefinable supplement which may make us whole again. Erotic desire thus may be triggered by rather specific bodily features, and we may invest our libido in particular parts of beloved bodies that are valued as particularly fascinating and intriguing. This may involve body parts such as breasts, phalluses, eyes, hands, muscles, buttocks or earlobes, although desire may also be aroused by the other's voice, gaze or smile, or even by specific ornaments or garments (such as high heels or pearl earrings) as symbolic equivalents of partial organs. It is not in the beloved other *as such*, but rather in specific bodily parts (or their replacements) that lovers suddenly discern what they have been (unconsciously) looking for: the emblem of human perfection, the lost object of desire, which suddenly seems to resurge before their very eyes, which suddenly seems to be there, presenting itself to them, invitingly.

Lacan uses the term *object a* to refer to partial objects (breasts, hands, feet,[1] voices, etc.) that function as (lost) objects of desire. He expresses this with the help of an equation, the so-called matheme of desire, where $ represents the (divided, craving) subject (yearning for wholeness), while *a* refers to the desirable object (the missing piece or item), and $\Diamond$ represents desire as a function which operates in both directions, for the lover is both drawn towards and focussed on the enigmatic object of desire: $ $\Diamond$ *a*.

---

[1] In the novel *Gradiva*, analysed by Freud (1907/1941), desire is aroused by the singular shape and movement of the heroine's feet that suddenly come into view.

The partial object, as object of desire (object a), also plays a crucial role in art. Partial objects which in normal life tend to remain concealed, may certainly protrude and unexpectedly emerge and come into view. In a seminar on anxiety, Lacan (1962–1963/2004) discusses two examples of religious art in which mutilated bodies are depicted, two paintings by the Spanish Baroque artist Francisco de Zurbarán (1598–1664) representing female saints (martyrs), namely Saint Lucia, carrying her severed eye-balls on a plate, and Saint Agatha, carrying her severed breasts on a similar plate. These parts had been violently removed in the context of religious persecutions to which they had been subjected. In normal life, we see the gaze, the pupils, but not the eye-balls of the other, and we see the outward shape and nipple, but not the internal tissues of the breasts. Separated from the body, these organs constitute something rather "uncanny", as we have seen (Freud 1919/1947). Such uncanny iconic visualisations confirm a basic subliminal anxiety concerning the detachable nature of the items involved. As stand-alone objects, removed and alienated from the body, they become obscene exhibits: too visible, too obtrusive and too close-up to be beautiful.

For Lacan, the uncanny is not restricted to aesthetics, however. The concept may especially be employed to address experiences invoked by technologies that affect human embodiment, such as transplantation medicine or synthetic biology (Zwart 2012, 2014). Uncanny is a removable body part that becomes *too real*. All of a sudden, the object of desire (the object a) becomes a "partial object", disconcerting rather than alluring.[2] Something similar goes for hands, or intestines, or even the complete skin, as in the case of Saint Bartholomew, or any other organ that is violently separated from the body as a whole. To use another Lacanian formula, the integrity of the body (A) is fundamentally damaged ($Ⱥ$). Its dignity and wholeness (1) must somehow be restored through the recovery of (and reconnection with) this object a, so that $Ⱥ + a = 1$.

---

[2] In an intriguing analysis, Iris Marian Young (1992) juxtaposes "breastedness" with mastectomy, building on the work of Luce Irigaray (a critical follower of Lacan). In Western patriarchal culture, dominated by the masculine gaze, she argues, women's breasts easily become objectified into a fetish that can be handled, manipulated, even "owned" by males as an object which is detachable from her body, functioning as "object of exchange" on the market of sexuality. This latent detachability is exemplified by breast removal in the case of malignancy, resulting in a breast-less or one-breasted (Amazon) woman, who may replace her missing breast with a prosthesis, thus underscoring its apparent replaceability.

Besides as objects of desire, however, partial objects may also serve as targets of aggression and appropriation. Here, cannibalism (as a cultural bodily practice documented by ethnographers/cultural anthropologists) stands out as an archetypal exemplification.

REFERENCES

Freud, S. 1907/1941. Der Wahn und die Träume in W. Jensens *Gradiva*. In *Gesammelte Werke VII*, 29–122. London: Imago.

———. 1919/1947. Das Unheimliche. In *Gesammelte Werke XII*, 227–268. London: Imago.

Lacan, J. 1962–1963/2004. *Le Séminaire de Jacques Lacan X: L'Angoisse*. Paris: Éditions du Seuil.

Young, I.M. 1992. Breasted Experience: The Look and the Feeling. In *The Body in Medical Thought and Practice*, Philosophy & Medicine, ed. Drew Leder, vol. 43, 215–230. Dordrecht/Boston/London: Kluwer.

Zwart, H. 2012. On Decoding and Rewriting Genomes: A Psychoanalytical Reading of a Scientific Revolution. *Medicine, Healthcare and Philosophy: A European Journal* 15 (3): 337–346.

———. 2014. The Donor Organ as an 'Object A': A Lacanian Perspective on Organ Donation and Transplantation Medicine. *Medicine, Health Care & Philosophy: A European Journal* 17 (4): 559–571. https://doi.org/10.1007/s11019-014-9553-1.

CHAPTER 6

Cannibalism and the Partial Object

Abstract Another body practice, focussed on specific body parts as objects of desire, is cannibalism. What is eaten in cannibalism is not the body of another person as such. Specific organs are singled out for consumption, associated with specific psychic features, personality traits which man-eaters may wish to incorporate. Specific parts or organs are literally incorporated to enhance particular virtues or to remedy particular deficit. We will consider why organ procurement has been explicitly compared to cannibalism in contemporary discourse.

Keywords Cannibalism • Partial objects • Matheme of desire • Incorporation • Human dignity

Cannibalism[1] (anthropophagy) is the harvesting of bodily parts or organs from cadavers after battle, the posthumous procurement of organs by victorious others. What is eaten in cannibalism is not the body of another person as such. Specific organs are singled out for consumption, associated with specific psychic features, personality traits which man-eaters may wish to incorporate through cannibalism—for example, courage by eating the

---

[1] *Caníbales* was the Spanish name for the Carib people of the West Indies, notorious for their cannibalistic practices. Cannibalism is used here not to refer to man-eating as a last resort to fend off starvation, such as occurred during the infamous Andes flight disaster in 1972, but as a ritualistic event notably practised by warriors and priests.

© The Author(s) 2019
H. A. E. Zwart, *Purloined Organs,*
https://doi.org/10.1007/978-3-030-05354-3_6

heart of a slain courageous enemy. In his ethnography classic *The Golden Bough*—a document which had a profound influence on psychoanalysis, notably on the work of Freud—Sir James Frazer (1890/1993) emphasised that cannibalism (once widespread) had always been a highly symbolic practice. Referring to a Central African tribe, bent on consuming specific organs harvested from the corpses of adversaries of favourable repute, he writes for instance:

> The flesh and blood of dead men are eaten and drunk to inspire bravery, wisdom or other qualities for which the men themselves were remarkable, or which are supposed to have their special seat in the particular part eaten ... Whenever an enemy who has behaved with conspicuous bravery is killed, his liver, which is considered the seat of valour; his ears, which are supposed to be the seat of intelligence; the skin of his forehead, which is regarded as the seat of perseverance; his testicles, which are held to be the seat of strength; and other members, which are viewed as the seat of other virtues, are cut from his body, baked to cinders and ... mixed with other ingredients into a kind of paste. (p. 497)

Thus, flesh coming from humans is not regarded as food. Rather, specific parts or organs are "incorporated" to enhance particular virtues, or to remedy particular deficits ($Å + a = 1$).

These ideas were taken up by Freud: by consuming specific body parts of defeated foes, particular characteristics were literally "incorporated", he argued. Cannibalism is not primarily about food. It is about identification with the (idealised) other (1913/1940, p. 101, 172, 1905/1942, p. 98, 1921/1940, p. 116, 1923/1940, p. 257). A surplus of strength or courage is added by procuring and consuming specific organs (singled out by particular theories of localisation). It is not the body as such which is consumed, but certain favoured parts. The cannibalistic desire may focus on partial objects such as heart, ears and testicles: components which are set apart as especially valuable. What the man-eater is after is a particular organ, hidden inside the other's body, brought to the surface, ready for the harvest. In other words, the cannibal strides to battle guided by the Lacanian formula: $ \$ \Diamond a $.[2]

---

[2] In Shakespeare's *The Merchant of Venice*, a similar formula is at work: the heart is set apart from the rest of the body and the question is how to collect the heart as something which can be surgically separated from the remaining bodily *real*.

In contemporary culture, cannibalism (although not formally listed among the psychiatric conditions mentioned in the *Diagnostic and Statistical Manual of Mental Disorders*) is associated with serial killers and considered a sexual perversion. A famous (albeit fictional) contemporary devotee is Hannibal Lecter, a former psychoanalyst and art connoisseur who becomes a wanted cannibalistic killer in a series of well-known movies. His object *a* may be the face of his victims, ripping the flesh off their faces with his bare teeth, but he may also go for the intestines (as happens in the case of the unfortunate police inspector Rinaldo Pazzi, whose disembowelled body is hung from the balcony of the Palazzo della Signoria in Florence) or for the brain (as in the case of justice department official Paul Krendler, whose skull is lifted so that parts of his brain can be eaten for lunch). Lecter's intentionality (as a craving subject: $) becomes fixated on a particular part of the victim's body. His desire adheres to the formula $ ◊ a.

Although the analogy between the procurement of cadaveric organs for transplantation and cannibalism may seem far-fetched, a structural similarity can nonetheless be discerned. Organ procurement has been explicitly compared to cannibalism by a number of authors, including Leon Kass (1992). In a provocative paper, he endeavours to analyse the (unconscious) origins of his uneasiness with transplantation medicine. How can I, he asks himself, see organ donation (involving a life-saving gift to a lethally suffering patient) as an "unsavoury practice"? What is the cause of the resistance? The paper amounts to an exercise in auto-analysis by a self-questioning ethicist who puts himself on the couch (Zwart 2016). What is so impelling about organ transplantation, Kass concludes, is that the body is treated as "a heap of alienable spare parts" (1992, p. 66), which undermines the body's dignity. Due to the technical possibility of salvaging organs, the human body has become a valuable resource of materials which we should not allow to go wasted, which should not be left unused. Therefore, "organ transplantation really is—once we strip away the trappings of sterile operating rooms and their astonishing technologies—simply a noble form of cannibalism" (p. 73).[3]

---

[3] In this same vein, voyeurism is defined by Kass (1992) as "cannibalism of the eyes".

REFERENCES

Frazer, J. 1890/1993. *The Golden Bough*. London: Wordsworth.

Freud, S. 1905/1942. Drei Abhandlungen zur Sexualtheorie. In *Gesammelte Werke V*, 27–145. London: Imago.

———. 1913/1940. Totem und Tabu. In *Gesammelte Werke IX*. London: Imago.

———. 1921/1940. Massenpsychologie und Ich-Analyse. In *Gesammelte Werke XIII*, 71–162. London: Imago.

———. 1923/1940. Das Ich und das Es. In *Gesammelte Werke XIII*, 237–289. London: Imago.

Kass, L. 1992. Organs for Sale? Propriety, Property, and the Price of Progress. *The Public Interest* Spring (107): 65–86.

Zwart, H. 2016. Psychoanalysis and Bioethics: A Lacanian Approach to Bioethical Discourse. *Medicine, Healthcare and Philosophy* 19 (4): 605–621. https://doi.org/10.1007/s11019-016-9698-1.

CHAPTER 7

Another Analogy: The Catholic Devotion to the Sacred Heart

Abstract Another cultural practice which shares resemblances with donation, and which may therefore be regarded as a precursor of organ transplantation medicine, is the Catholic devotion to the Sacred Heart of Christ. This devotion acts out a basic ambivalence that runs through Christianity as far as the body is concerned. On the one hand, Christianity emphatically commits itself to understanding human embodiment in terms of inviolability, unity and integrity. This poses obstacles to transplantation medicine, notably to salvaging cadaveric organs for transplantation. On the other hand, there is the contrasting idea of charity and love, the attitude of self-sacrifice, as exemplified by the devotion of the Sacred Heart.

Keywords Sacred Heart • Christianity • Resurrection • Inviolability • Sharing • Donation

Another cultural practice which bears resemblances to donation, and which may therefore be regarded as a precursor of organ transplantation medicine, is the Catholic devotion to the Sacred Heart of Christ. This devotion can be seen as an acting-out of a basic ambivalence that runs through Christianity as far as the body is concerned. On the one hand, Christianity has emphatically committed itself to understanding human embodiment in terms of inviolability, unity and integrity as we have seen.

This poses serious obstacles to transplantation medicine, notably to salvaging cadaveric organs for transplantation (Zwart and Hoffer 1998). One is not allowed to use or recycle the bodies of deceased persons, nor is one entitled to violate their bodily integrity. Piety towards human corpses has been instilled and imprinted by Christianity into Western culture throughout the ages and has solidified into deep-seated moral intuitions. Indeed, in late Roman and early medieval times, Christian propaganda effectively put a stop to ritual practice such as incineration, replacing funeral pyres with graves. This was closely connected with the dogma of the resurrection of the body: on Resurrection Day, when the trumpet calls (as Saint Paul phrases it),[1] body and soul will be reunited into a transfigured, imperishable body and for that reason, the integrity of the body has to be preserved, even posthumously—although the widespread practice of harvesting relics from bodies of deceased Saints may seem at odds with this principle of post-mortal inviolability.

On the other hand, there is the contrasting idea of charity and love (in the sense of *agape*), the attitude of self-sacrifice, as exemplified by the devotion of the Sacred Heart. During the Last Supper, Christ shared His own flesh and blood with His disciples.[2] In pictorial renderings of the devotion to the Sacred Heart, the love (i.e. the willingness to share, care and give) of Christ has become so overwhelmingly great that His heart almost seems to rise to the surface of His body. His (wounded) heart becomes visible, as if a kind of window is opened up, providing access into His thorax, which has become transparent, under the sway of burning compassion. What is usually hidden, within the *camera obscura* of our body, suddenly protrudes, becoming visible and touchable. From the profundity of His chest, His sharing love radiates into the world. Christ is offering His heart to suffering individuals; it has become the sublime object *a* par excellence, the thing that may sooth our yearning desires, our tormenting deficiencies. Indeed, the very thing that we (as devotees) were (unconsciously) seeking, now suddenly reveals itself, in a phantasmagorical fashion. A similar experience may befall patients who are suddenly told that a donor kidney or liver is available at last. This tension between a duty

---

[1] "The trumpet shall sound, and the dead shall be raised incorruptible, and we shall be changed" (1 Corinthians 15:52).

[2] Indeed, the Last Supper, and the sacrament of the communion (conducted behind closed doors) which builds on it, has been regarded as a (sublimated) remnant of cannibalism by critics of Christianity notably in Roman times.

to safeguard bodily integrity on the one hand and the eagerness to share and give, introduces a normative split in Christian morality at a very fundamental level. The compromise position is to regard organ donation as something which may solely be practised as a gift. From a Christian perspective, the commodification of organ donation (the idea of organs for sale) incites moral repugnance. From a liberal perspective, however, this repugnance is regarded as irrational, and as an obstacle to the development of an organ market to solve the scarcity issues of organ transplant medicine (Erin and Harris 2003; Zwart and Hoffer 1998).

References

Erin, C., and J. Harris. 2003. An Ethical Market in Human Organs. *Journal of Medical Ethics* 29: 137–138.

Zwart, H., and C. Hoffer. 1998. *Orgaandonatie en lichamelijke integriteit*. Best: Damon.

CHAPTER 8

Types of Discourse

Abstract Psychoanalytically speaking, in the organ transplantation debate, various types of discourse can be distinguished, each of them conveying a logic of its own. In this chapter, their discursive profiles and specificities will be outlined, building on Lacan's theorem of the four discourses. Whereas the hysteric's discourse gives the floor the tormented subject who raises a voice of protest against the establishment, the discourse of the Master is devoted to explaining and sustaining a particular authoritative view of human embodiment. In university discourse, the qualified expert takes the floor, representing biomedical or bioethical expertise. Finally, the discourse of the analyst revolves around the question of why procurable organs have become objects of desire and how this affects embodied experience and subjectivity.

Keywords Four discourses • Discourse of the Master • University discourse • Hysteric's discourse • Discourse of the analyst • Biomedical discourse • Bioethical discourse • Divided subject

In the previous chapters, various types of discourse have been consulted, each of them conveying a logic of its own. In this chapter, their discursive profiles and specificities will be outlined more precisely, building on Lacan's theorem of the *four discourses* (Lacan 1969–1970/1991; cf. Zwart 2016, 2017). First of all, we have consulted forms of discourse which are

© The Author(s) 2019
H. A. E. Zwart, *Purloined Organs*,
https://doi.org/10.1007/978-3-030-05354-3_8

guided by an authoritative (allegedly unquestionable) source of insight, truth and knowledge, such as *Genesis* (attributed to Moses), or the works of Aristotle, or the *Epistles* of Saint Paul. *Genesis*, for instance, articulates the guiding idea that human beings were created in the image and likeness of God (*Genesis* 1:27). And Saint Paul, as we have seen, presents the body as an inviolable whole (wherein its dignity resides). This same conviction also functions as a starting point for the portrayal of the human body in Paradise by Thomas Aquinas, outlined earlier. In this type of discourse, *Genesis* or *Aristotle* is regarded as an indisputable, primary source, the legacy of an authoritative author: the primary subject of discourse (in Lacanian algebra: S_1). The recipients of the message are expert readers (from medieval scholars up to contemporary author experts) who see themselves as custodians of a legacy and whose writings are basically comments and interpretations (S_2). Lacan refers to this type of discourse as the *discourse of the Master*. It can be represented with the formula $S_1 \rightarrow S_2$. The Master addresses his followers/disciples, who are thus enabled to constitute themselves as experts, by carefully studying the authoritative source.

The scientific revolution entailed a dramatic shift in orientation, however. Experts (S_2) now emancipate themselves, taking the floor as autonomous researchers, as *agents*, driven by the resolve not to rely on the authority of others (S_1), but to produce knowledge themselves, by interacting with the world (the object) directly, in an *active* manner, through experimental research for instance, with the help of technical equipment and professional skills. Even the Bible becomes an *object* of research (rather than an authoritative source). This also applies to biomedical research. Professional experts (S_2) no longer rely on Aristotle or Hippocrates (S_1) and they no longer see themselves as disciples of a Master (as someone who *knows*), but explore the human body themselves as independent researchers, such as Vesalius, for instance, who disclosed the fabric of the body with his scalpel, replacing Bible reading by empirical inquiry, relying on technological skills rather than on authoritative texts, focussing on the body's basic components (bones, muscles, sinews, etc.). A more recent example is Karl Landsteiner (discussed earlier) who explored the basic components of blood cells, notably the antigens as enigmatic objects (benign and indispensable, but also potentially toxic, as fleshed out in Stoker's novel *Dracula*), enabling the identification of blood types. This results in a new type of discourse, referred to by Lacan as *university discourse*, whose structure concurs with the formula $S_2 \rightarrow a$. The biomedical experts (S_2) direct their questions to the enigmatic object (a) directly, without consulting Aristotle first. In the case of transplantation medicine, professional intentionality is focussed on an enigmatic, allusive "something" which proves difficult to procure and, once implanted, remains an object of concern: both life-saving and toxic, both intrusive and benign (the transplant organ as object a).

A third type of discourse emerges when neither the authoritative Master (Aristotle, Hippocrates, etc.: S_1), nor the scholarly or biomedical expert (S_2), but the patient herself or himself enters the scene and takes the floor, for instance via newspaper interviews, or autobiographical memoirs or personal blogs. Patients may produce ego-documents to verbalise their experiences as recipients or donors,[1] as tormented subjects ($\$$), driven by desire, but dependent on the medical establishment, desperate but also mistrustful. The voice of the tormented subject notably takes the floor to address and challenge reluctant authorities: those who try to limit organ recycling by referring to the integrity and the inviolability of the body for instance ($\$ \rightarrow S_1$). Lacan refers to this type of discourse as the *hysteric's discourse*.

The final type of discourse is the *discourse of the analyst*, revolving around the following question: what is it that tormented subjects (patients, but also biomedical researchers) really want? What kind of object is the transplant organ (the object a), and why has it become such an object of desire, not only for patients, but also for scientific researchers, calling them into action, forcing them to spend (or waste) years of their lives on efforts to tame and domesticate the object a? This type of discourse concurs with the formula $a \rightarrow \$$.

These formulas can be inserted into a quadruped scheme (Fig. 8.1).

This procedure results in four types of discourse, representable by four discursive quadrupeds (Fig. 8.2).

In the *discourse of the Master*, the credibility of the Master (S_1) is indisputable, as we have seen: there is no room for uncertainty and doubt ($\$$ is pushed into the lower-left position). Although in real life the Master may have been besieged by questions and anomalies, his disciples consider his teachings as unquestionable, revering him as the one who apodictically teaches truth.

Fig. 8.1 Lacan's quadruped scheme

Agent	Other
Disavowed truth	By-product

[1] The Dutch novelist A.H.J. Dautzenberg (2011) published a book entitled *Samaritan* about his decision to volunteer as a kidney donor.

Discourse of the Master		University discourse	
S_1	S_2	S_2	a
$\$$	a	S_1	$\$$

Discourse of the hysteric		Discourse of the analyst	
$\$$	S_1	a	$\$$
a	S_2	S_2	S_1

Fig. 8.2   The four discourses

In *university discourse*, however (and in biomedical discourse as a special branch of university discourse), the voice of the Master (S_1) is silenced and repressed (pushed into the lower-left position), so that this type of discourse is allegedly neutral and objective. Religious or ideological convictions have been pushed aside. On closer inspection, however, ideologies are still at work, as we have seen (from below the bar). Biomedical discourse (more specifically: transplantation medicine) is inspired by *and* propagates a basic view of embodiment, a basic *philosopheme* (S_1), although it requires a "depth" ethics to bring this to the surface. Transplantation medicine abolishes the image of the inviolable body and replaces it with a rival idea: the body as an aggregate of replaceable parts (S_1). A special type of university discourse is bioethical discourse (e.g. Den Hartogh 2013a, 2013b), bent on developing a normative conceptual infrastructure to facilitate the procurement and transplantation of human organs. Again, it is a type of discourse which tends to present itself as metaphysically neutral, as non-ideological and so on, but on closer inspection it conveys a very specific view of embodiment (S_1): the body as an aggregate of reusable parts, combined with a particular (neo-liberal) understanding of the subject, namely as an autonomous person and as the "owner" of this body (Zwart and Hoffer 1998).

Hysterics challenge traditional authorities, as we have seen. They tend to experience their bodies as dismembered and deficient ($\$$), suffering from a lack which can allegedly be sutured by organ transplantation, with the help of a partial object. This object arouses their desire, but also their mistrustfulness, for the object a is something which is both life-saving and toxic, both enabling and paralysing. A weakness of this type of discourse, from a Lacanian perspective, is that these divided subjects ($) in the position of the agent do not really know what is driving them; they do not really know what they want. It requires a clock-wise turn to the right (the discourse of the analyst) to reveal the *agency* of the object: its alluring and seducing qualities, which, in the discourse of the hysteric, tend to be disavowed (pushed into the lower-left position). In the discourse of the analyst, expert knowledge is being suspended (S_2 pushed into the lower-left position), so that the focus shifts towards the patient as a *recipient* (a subject of desire: $), called upon by an alluring but potentially disruptive object (a) calling out to him or her.

To every type of discourse, moreover, there is a by-product (lower-right position). Although Christianity celebrates the inviolable body (S_1), it produces the devotion of the Sacred Heart as we have seen, staged as a gesture of sharing a partial organ (a). And although university discourse is bent on control (aspiring to domesticate the object a), the experiment may dramatically falter, resulting in despair (among recipients or their surgeons), for instance, when transplant organs are rejected, so that, rather than live-saving, they become intrusive and toxic, items of concern, to such an extent perhaps that organ transplantation medicine is experienced as an impossible endeavour ($). In mainstream bioethical discourse, patients are staged as autonomous decision-makers (i.e. agents), while the object tends to be portrayed in a purely instrumental manner, as an item which can be domesticated and transformed into a means to an end, something which saves lives and restores an ailing body to normalcy or health. The recalcitrance of the implanted organ and, as a consequence of that, the suffering of patients ($), whose implants are rejected, emerge as unexpected by-products. In the upcoming chapters, we will further elaborate this overview of the four discourses as we proceed.

After this methodological intermezzo, I will now return to the problem of organs as commodities. Having discussed commodification from a Christian and a Kantian perspective (earlier), in the next chapter the focus will shift to how this issue is thematised by Lacan.

REFERENCES

Dautzenberg, A.H.J. 2011. *Samaritaan*. Amsterdam/Antwerp: Contact.
Den Hartogh, G. 2013a. Is Consent of the Donor Enough to Justify the Removal of Living Organs? *Cambridge Quarterly of Healthcare Ethics* 22 (1): 45–54.

————. 2013b. The Political Obligation to Donate Organs. *Ratio Juris* 26 (3): 378–403.

Lacan, J. 1969–1970/1991. *Le séminaire XVII: L'envers de la psychanalyse*. Paris: Éditions du Seuil.

Zwart, H. 2016. Psychoanalysis and Bioethics: A Lacanian Approach to Bioethical Discourse. *Medicine, Healthcare and Philosophy* 19 (4): 605–621. https://doi.org/10.1007/s11019-016-9698-1.

————. 2017. *Tales of Research Misconduct: A Lacanian Diagnostics of Integrity Challenges in Science Novels*. Library of Ethics and Applied Philosophy. Cham: Springer. https://doi.org/10.1007/978-3-319-65554-3.

Zwart, H., and C. Hoffer. 1998. *Orgaandonatie en lichamelijke integriteit*. Best: Damon.

CHAPTER 9

Commodification of Organs As Objects of Desire

Abstract Building on Marx and Freud, Lacan reflects on how commodities become objects of desire. The commodity becomes a fetish, a replacement of a partial object (the object of desire). This raises the question about what happens if organs themselves become commodities, procurable on the organ market, allegedly representing the one thing suffering subjects desperately need. Transplantation medicine emerges as a technological development with decisive ontological repercussions.

Keywords Commodification • Marxism • Organs as commodities • Objects of desire • Sublimation • Phantasmagoria

The commodification of objects of desire became an important theme for Lacan, notably in the seminars which he presented during the late 1960s: the era of leftist student revolts, in Paris and elsewhere. In this context, besides building on Freud, he often cites and consults the commodification theory developed by Karl Marx (1867/1979). In this chapter, I will flesh out the conceptual building blocks of Lacan's problematisation of commodities. As indicated, his theories first and foremost lean on Freud but are further elaborated in confrontation with the political-economical views of Marx—which were quite in vogue at that time, and the core focus of attention of his friend Louis Althusser (Althusser and Balibar 1970).

© The Author(s) 2019
H. A. E. Zwart, *Purloined Organs*,
https://doi.org/10.1007/978-3-030-05354-3_9

In the subsequent chapter (Chap. 10), these views will be extrapolated towards organ transplantation medicine as a praxis.

In *Capital* (1867/1979), Marx explains how workers, as soon as they enter the industrial labour market, are duped by capitalists, who face them with a "sardonic grin" (Lacan 1968–1969/2006, p. 65). They receive less than they produce because they are bereft of the surplus value of their labour. They become estranged from the products they actually produced themselves, notably when these products enter the market as commodities. As commodities on display, industrial products acquire a mystical, "phantasmagorical" (1867/1979, p. 86), even "fetish"-like (p. 87) character, Marx argues. To reframe it in Lacanian terms (1968–1969/2006, pp. 16–18), rather than simply being useful entities which may satisfy bodily needs, they become *objects of desire.*

The term fetish is aptly chosen because commodities (on display in a shop window or an advertisement, for instance) should not be conceived as passive or neutral entities. Rather, they are connected with bodies and body parts (partial organs) in various ways. Consumables may incite oral enticements (EAT ME, DRINK ME, as *Alice in Wonderland* phrases it), unleashing oral desire: a craving that goes beyond the mere satisfaction of biological needs. Certain commodities (certain brands of wine or whiskey, for instance) promise singular forms of satisfaction, which the usual products fail to provide. Mattresses, cushions and beds may promise more than merely keeping us warm at night. They may purport to create optimal conditions for erotic pleasure. A bed may simply be a bed (a useful thing), but it may also become a site of primal scenes: the marriage bed where life begins, intimate relationships are consumed and children are conceived and delivered. Other items (such as hammers or motorbikes) may suggest enhanced strength and swiftness, upgraded "phallic" performance. Still others (such as toothbrushes or bath tubs) suggest options for corporeal cleansing and hygiene (the "anal" dimension). Cell phones and CDs may convey the promise of connecting us with the *voice* of the Other, while laptops and tablets may be exceptionally tempting insofar as they promise to connect us with the *gaze* of the Other, allowing the alluring object to enter our *stage*, our *field of vision*, our fantasy-world, as a captivating Gestalt. Finally, inviting images of white beaches and blue lagoons may convey hints of experiences of *jouissance* which we (unconsciously) long for, but which are normally withheld from us. This is how commodities (as objects of desire) speak to us: they enter our life-world by connecting objects with (unconscious) desires. And this explains their phantasmagorical, fetish-like aura: they convey the promise that (after extended periods of hard work) dreams may finally come true. The commodity purports to bridge the gap between labour and pleasure. Objects from which the labourers became estranged (in the course of the production process) suddenly show up in a commercial, as alluring objects of desire. The pleasure which was renounced during productivity (the hard work of industrial labour) is suddenly retrieved: encapsulated in commodities.

Freud emphasises, moreover, that commodities (as objects of desire) may mimic certain bodily functions, a process he refers to as *Anlehnung*. The commodity reflects and builds on the functioning of a partial organ, so that the desire becomes *displaced* (*verschoben*) from the partial organ to a (technologically reproducible) substitute. Although a commodity is allegedly decontextualised (disconnected from the intimacy of the body), the absent (disconnected) body part is nonetheless still implicated. Insofar as alluring commodities reflect our bodily desires, the next question is: what happens if organs *themselves* become commodities or things for sale? What happens when organs (partial objects) become procurable as market products? What kind of thing or commodity are they?

A first outline of an answer is provided by Freud in his essay *The uncanny* ("Das Unheimliche", 1919/1947), already briefly discussed earlier, where he argues that partial organs (such as eyes, for instance), separated from the body (as detachable and replaceable parts), are bound to strike us as uncanny, that is, as both fascinating and repelling. The uncanny is that which seems familiar and alienating at the same time, that which should have remained hidden, but is suddenly revealed. The experience of the uncanny indicates that items which are intimately known may suddenly become disconcerting, as stand-alone objects. This seems a fitting description of the experiences evoked by undead organs as living things, procured from brain-dead bodies and placed in a bowl filled with ice. In the next chapter, I will point out how these insights, borrowed from Marx and Freud, are taken up by Lacan, whose seminars (conducted from 1953 up to 1978) coincided with the first (decisive) decades of transplantation medicine.

References

Althusser, L., and E. Balibar. 1970. *Lire le capital*. Paris: Maspero.

Freud, S. 1919/1947. Das Unheimliche. In *Gesammelte Werke XII*, 227–268. London: Imago.

Lacan, J. 1968–1969/2006. *Le Séminaire de Jacques Lacan XVI: D'un Autre à l'autre*. Paris: Éditions du Seuil.

Marx, K. 1867/1979. *Das Kapital. Kritik der politischen Oekonomie 1: der produktionsprocess des Kapitals*. Berlin: Dietz.

CHAPTER 10

A Lacanian Assessment of Organ Transplantation

Abstract Due to transplantation medicine, the procurable organ becomes an object of desire: that which purports to make us whole again, set apart and standing out from the rest of the body of the other, from which the organ is harvested, as an entity in its own right—the one thing we desire more than anything else, that which may compensate our deficiencies, our deprivations, making our destitute body whole again. Lacan explains how the faltering organ creates a sense of emptiness (a vacuole) which the procurable, transplantable organ claims to fill, as something both foreign and intimate, both life-saving and toxic: as an "extimate" object.

Keywords Fragmentation • Trauma • Displacement • The uncanny • Organ replacement • Vacuole • Extimacy

In everyday experience, human beings tend to perceive their body as an integrated whole: we basically experience wholeness. Various sections of our body are regarded as part and parcel of what we as *individuals* (literally, "indivisible beings") are. Wholeness therefore seems a primary experience, preceding our awareness of specific organs within the body. On closer inspection, however, this is questionable. Lacan points out, as we have seen, that our primary experience is rather one of fragmentation, where the divide between internal and external, self and other is decidedly unclear. The experience of bodily wholeness is a temporary and fragile outcome of an interminable dialectical process of incorporation and separation, starting with the trauma of birth. Moreover, experiences of bodily wholeness may be dramatically undermined in cases of illness.[1] When specific organs (heart, lungs, kidneys) or other constituents (joints, bones, tissues, etc.) suddenly fail, they stand out, as it were, from the body as a (wholesome) whole. The failing or faltering part becomes a focus of attention, and may even become an obsession, while at the same time providing a point of access (a window into the intimacy of the body) for processes of symbolisation, via intrusive biomedical technologies. Because of the affected organ, the body becomes subjected to measurements and inquiries. High-tech contrivances bring the faltering organ into view, comparing its dysfunctionality with functionality, its quantifiable performance with normal values (normalcy). Should the disrupted/disruptive organ endanger the well-being of the body as a whole, removal may be considered as an option and the body becomes an aggregate/composite of organs. If other treatment options fail, one of our organs may be expelled or even become a candidate for replacement.

From that point onwards, attention may turn towards the bodies of others: potential donors; not to their bodies *as such*, but to specific parts (a kidney, a cornea, a uterus,[2] etc.). Intentionality becomes focussed on a *partial object* encased within the bodies of others. A specific organ becomes an object of desire: an object *a*, which purports to make us whole again, set apart from the rest of the bodies of these others, an entity in its own right—the one thing we desire more than anything else ($ \$ \lozenge a $), the one thing that may compensate our deficiency, our deprivation, by making our destitute body whole again ($ \cancel{A} + a = 1 $).

The transplant, although being an organ, is not a natural entity moreover. It is an artefact of transplantation medicine, made available by technical developments, and also (in the case of cadaveric organs) by legal constructs such as the brain-death concept, in combination with a donor's will and other symbolic conditions. It is a rather intractable thing that may be either present or absent, available or non-available, depending on bio-

---

[1] Freud already pointed this out: "Die Pathologie lehrt uns eine große Anzahl von Zuständen kennen, in denen die Abgrenzung des Ichs gegen die Außenwelt unsicher wird… Fälle in denen uns Teile des eigenen Körpers… wie fremd und dem Ich nicht zugehörig erscheinen" (1930/1948, p. 423; cf. above).

[2] http://www.cbsnews.com/news/nine-swedish-women-undergo-uterus-transplants/.

medical supplies and tissue matching, but also on codicils and various other factors that affect the viability and legitimacy of the act of transplantation.

If we place ourselves in the position of the donor, we may discern in the suffering Other (the potential recipient) a gap or lack, a deficit we are called upon to fill with our gift, either as a living donor or, after (brain) death, as a cadaver, via organ procurement. As Lacan phrases it, in one of his seminars, these suffering others utter an inaudible *scream*, like the one depicted in a famous series of paintings produced by Edvard Munch bearing this title, awaiting the arrival of someone who may fill the gap and ease the discontent (1968–1969/2006, p. 225).

Inside the body of the suffering Other, an anatomical emptiness may be discerned: a gap, which Lacan refers to as a "vacuole" (1968–1969/2006, p. 232), a term which usually applies to the anatomy of unicellular organisms, but is used here to indicate this ambiguous, sinister, empty space that was once occupied by a now dysfunctional or dispelled organ. This space can only be filled by a gift from the Other, by an object *a*.

Tissue matching and immune-repressive drugs, in combination with informed consent procedures, will determine the extent to which organs are actually available and transferable from one body to another. This involves measurements and calculations: a drastic symbolisation of the body and its tissues, as well as a barrage of legal procedures. The objective is to restore the recipient's body to *normality* (a symbolic concept, describable in terms of quantifiable indicators) rather than *integrity* (a concept which refers to the imaginary view of the body in terms of wholeness and therefore belongs to the realm of the "ideal", as Lacan points out: 2006, p. 270). Normality rather than integrity is the goal. In fact, the integrity of the body, in the form of the immune system, will offer resistance and may even "reject" the implanted organ. Much effort will be spent in counteracting this natural response of the body as a whole. Organ implantation leaves considerable scars: the integrity of the body is partially restored, but also damaged forever, by the intrusive act of implantation and everything this entails (invasive surgery, immune-repressive drugs, the introduction of foreign tissue, the brutal scars of the operation, etc.).[3]

---

[3] Lacan also makes a connection with perversion. The perverse subject discerns that something is missing in the body of the other (for instance, the phallus). This is represented as $Ⱥ$, the barred Other, who falls short of the imaginary ideal. This deficiency has to be restored with the help of a certain supplement, an equivalent for the missing object *a*, so that the Other can be brought back to his/her level of dignity again: $Ⱥ + a = 1$ (2006, p. 19).

Thus, there is first of all an intimate gap within the recipient's body, a vacuole, as Lacan phrases it, which cries out to us, and wherein the donated organ is to be implanted. A gift from an Other is inserted into this empty space. To explain what is entailed in this event, and to articulate the (weird, ambiguous) ontological status of the implanted organ, Lacan introduces the term "extimate": a portmanteau word, blending two concepts, namely *external* and *intimate*, into one neologism, emphasising the paradoxical nature of organ donation. The body's intimate interior is opened up, its integrity is disrespected and an implant is inserted: something which is both intimate and external, both self and other, both familiar and foreign—an *extimate* object. The new organ will remain a precarious thing, an object of concern, and may never become wholly embedded once and for all. It may never become a completely integrated part of the body. As an "extimate" object, it is both eerily strange and profoundly intimate: toxic and benevolent, fragile and highly vulnerable, a concern for life.[4] Extimacy implies that the object, while being on the inside, remains stigmatised and different: an ambiguous thing of whose presence and performance the recipient remains acutely aware.[5] Extimacy stresses that, due to transplantation medicine, the distance (the divide) between Self and Other dramatically decreases, while at the same time otherness remains, but now as something intimate and internal.

References

Bracher, M., M. Alcorn, F. Massardier-Kennedy, and R. Corthell, eds. 1994. *Lacanian Theory of Discourse: Subject, Structure, and Society*. New York: New York University Press.

Freud, S. 1930/1948. Das Unbehagen in der Kultur. In *Gesammelte Werke XIV*, 419–513. London: Imago.

Lacan, J. 1968–1969/2006. *Le Séminaire de Jacques Lacan XVI: D'un Autre à l'autre*. Paris: Éditions du Seuil.

---

[4] "J'ai désigné comme la *vacuole*, cet interdit au centre, qui constitue, en somme, ce qui nous est. le plus prochain, tout en nous étant extérieur. Il faudrait faire le mot *extime* pour désigner ce dont il s'agit" (2006, p. 224).

[5] The paradoxical concept of "extimacy" may been seen as comparable to Saint Augustine's famous phrase envisioning God as "interior intimo meo", more interior than my innermost being (Bracher et al. 1994, p. 76). The new organ is inside the recipient, but he/she remains highly aware of its presence.

CHAPTER 11

Alfred Adler's Concept of Organ Inferiority

Abstract To address the experience of faltering or deficient organs, Alfred Adler coined the term "organ inferiority". Organ inferiority refers to the human condition *as such*. Psychoanalytically speaking, we are *Mängelwesen* (deficient beings). Bodily deficiencies give rise to a chronic need for compensation, in the form of ersatz organs, which can only be provided by culture and technology. Yet, discontent resurges, as these ersatz organs entail physical and existential challenges of the own. Again, the question emerges how this works out when living organs present themselves as a replacement.

Keywords Organ inferiority • Mangelwesen • Competition • Compensation • Overcompensation

Although the work of Alfred Adler (1870–1937), one of the earliest "renegades" of the Freudian movement, is usually ignored by mainstream psychoanalysts, he actually devoted much attention to the (psychic) role and function of organs (1917/1927, 1927/2009). Therefore, his work deserves to be consulted in this context.

In psychoanalysis, as we have seen, the term "partial object" refers to a specific part of the body which can be seen as semi-separable. Precisely for this reason, partial objects such as penises or breasts may function as focus points during libidinal development. According to Freud, during the "oral stage" (the first 18 months of life), the mouth is the primary erogenous zone and the desire of young infants is focussed on breasts and nipples: body parts which may be absent or present, offered to us or denied to us, present in adult females but absent in males. Subsequently, during the "anal stage" (from 18 months to 3 years), the anus is the primary erogenous zone and excrements come to be seen as separable, detachable body parts. And finally, during the "phallic stage", the focus shifts to the phallus as a genital appendage whose presence or absence allows children to distinguish male from female. Thus, traditional Freudian psychoanalysis focuses on a limited set of partial organs.

This set was significantly expanded by Alfred Adler who coined the concept "organ inferiority" (Organminderwertigkeit). To a certain extent, organ inferiority refers to the human condition *as such*. We are, as Arnold Gehlen (1940/1962) once phrased it, *Mängelwesen*, and Adler adheres to this idea, seeing human feet, for instance, as stunted hands, and hands as stunted claws, and so forth. Bodily deficiencies give rise to a chronic need for compensation, which can only be provided by culture and technology. For instance, pyro-technology is developed to compensate for lack of fur. We are technology-dependent to a high degree because natural environments expect the organs of organisms to be fully up to their tasks, and with humans this is not the case. Even the human mind as such evolved as a protective organ to compensate for the lack of protection offered by other bodily parts and organs, thus evolving into our organ of adaptation par excellence.

Individuals who experience a particular type of organ inferiority will feel even more restrained and "curtailed" in comparison to others.[1] As a result, they aim to compensate their deficits, but this may well result in overcompensation, for example, when a child suffering from asthma becomes a top athlete in adult life. As Adler sees it, partial objects not only include breasts, penises and testicles (as in the traditional Freudian scheme), but also kidneys, lungs and muscles (Adler 1917/1927). While erotic desire tends to focus on a limited set of protruding organs (penises, breasts, earlobes, etc.), which we in principle could do without (in terms of mere survival), Adler puts more emphasis on organs that play a crucial role in physical survival (of humans as biological entities) and in our ability to come to terms with the competitiveness of modern societal existence:

---

[1] As Adler phrases it, organ inferiority gives rise to a sense of being disadvantaged: a *Gefühl der Verkürztheit*, which literally means a sense of being "shortened" (1927/2009).

organs involved in physiology, metabolism and mobility. Thus, organs such as lungs, heart and kidneys come into view as focal points for transplantation medicine. For the individuals involved, the inferior organ becomes an obsession, a shadow hovering over the narrative of their lives.

In Adler's work, the focus shifts from reproduction to survival and from *love* to *labour*, in the sense of professional performance and social competition. Organ deficiencies hamper social mobility and productivity, and individuals respond to this through compensation (or even overcompensation). Now that we have entered the era of transplantation medicine, organ and tissue transplantation may increasingly become a viable option in this respect: compensation through replacement. Instead of a life compromised by organ deficiency, an implant may enhance waning capacities, allowing us to become competitive again. Thus, partial organs become objects of desire for other reasons, not directly but indirectly related to erotic desire. There are other ways in which bodily parts may help us to overcome our sense of deficiency and lack.

Let this suffice as a presentation of our conceptual frame of reference. Now, the focus of attention will shift to case histories (representing the practical or empirical dimension of a psychoanalytical approach). In the next chapter, I will further elucidate the dialectical phenomenology of organ transplantation with the help of a first (unsettling) case history: the memoirs of Thomas Starzl (born in 1926), a prominent American transplantation pioneer. Thus, whereas in subsequent chapters the floor will be given to patients/recipients of transplant organs, I will start my practical ($N = 1$) analysis with an ego-document featuring a biomedical expert (a famous transplant surgeon) as *subject* of desire.

REFERENCES

Adler, A. 1917/1927. *Studie über Minderwertigkeit von Organen*. Darmstadt: Wissenschaftliche Buchgesellschaft.
———. 1927/2009. *Menschenkenntnis*. Frankfurt am Main: Fischer.
Gehlen, A. 1940/1962. *Der Mensch. Seine Natur und seine Stellung in der Welt*. Frankfurt: Athenäum.

CHAPTER 12

Thomas Starzl: A Case History

Abstract Case histories constitute a tested psychoanalytical technique for exploring experiential tensions, contradictions and ambivalences in a detailed manner. In this chapter, the memoirs of transplant surgeon Thomas Starzl are analysed. Starzl devoted his career to one particular partial object, the human liver. For Starzl, this organ stood out from the rest of the body as a surgical challenge par excellence: an enormous and silent reddish-brown organ that proved remarkably hostile to surgeons. The title of his memoirs (*"The puzzle people"*) echoes the idea that in the future, heart, liver and pancreas may really become replaceable, refurbishing the human body as an aggregate of replaceable parts. The acquisition of new parts requires that the rest of the body will have to change before the gift can be accepted. Indeed, even surgeons are profoundly changed by the impact of their experiences.

Keywords Thomas Starzl • Case studies • Rejection • Cyclosporine • Liver transplantation • Transplantation surgery

Case analysis is a tested psychoanalytical technique for exploring basic tensions, contradictions and ambivalences of human experience on a practical level. In this chapter, I will use the memoirs of transplant surgeon Thomas Starzl as a *Fallgeschichte*. Starzl devoted his whole career to one particular "partial object", his object *a*, the target of his *cupido sciendi*, namely the

© The Author(s) 2019
H. A. E. Zwart, *Purloined Organs,*
https://doi.org/10.1007/978-3-030-05354-3_12

human liver. For Starzl, this organ stood out from the rest of the body as a surgical challenge par excellence. When a human body is opened in a dissection room, the liver is what comes most prominently into view. This organ, which intrigued medicine since the dawn of anatomy, haunted Thomas Starzl for life. As he himself phrased it: "In seeking a purpose in life ... something at a subconscious level seemed to point to the liver ... an enormous and silent reddish-brown organ that had withheld many secrets of its own function and was hostile to surgeons" (Starzl 1992/2003, p. 54). The title of his memoirs ("*The puzzle people*") echoes a question by a journalist: "Do you think that in the next decade a puzzle man with a heart, liver and pancreas taken from other human beings might be feasible?" (p. 3). The metaphor captures the human body as an aggregate of replaceable parts in a truly Frankenstein fashion. As Starzl explains, however, the acquisition of new "parts" requires that the rest of the body will have to change before the gift can be accepted. Indeed, even surgeons are profoundly changed by the impact of their experiences (p. 4).

Starzl's father was editor of a local Iowa newspaper and author of science fiction stories about space travel and extra-terrestrial life. Starzl studied medicine in Chicago, where he had his first Frankensteinish experience:

> Dissatisfied with my knowledge of anatomy, I bought a cadaver of my own during my senior year... an Indian lady, not to be shared with other students. Late at night and on the weekends, I learned her body lovingly as if she were an old and dear friend, making amateur drawings as portions of her came off. She slowly disappeared. When she was gone, she had bequeathed me a knowledge of anatomy that I would carry for all my life. (p. 26)

A first step on his trajectory towards transplantation medicine was setting up a vessel bank, removing blood vessels from corpses in a Miami hospital morgue (p. 48), resulting in a first publication on transplantation issues. Subsequently he began to remove livers from dogs (hepatectomy) in a garage (as an improvised research facility), installing new livers "in the empty space from which the normal liver had been taken out" (p. 57)—in Lacanian terms, he artificially created "vacuoles" in the bodies of test animals for implantation purposes. These operations proved "far more difficult and bloody" than he had expected, however. In Lacanian terms, the *real* body remained a persistent obstacle. Repeated failure of liver transplants, first in dogs and subsequently in human patients, revealed a devastating conflict between the symbolic and the real body: between "medical dreams" and "harsh reality" (p. 63). His desire became to fathom the "mysterious" processes that destroy transplanted livers. He encountered the Real as a persistent, disruptive force, something unknown and uncanny that flouts our expectations, depriving a suffering body of its newly implanted organ. Gradually, it dawned on him that what was at work here was the active striving of the body itself to safeguard its integrity via its immune system. The patient's own body became the surgeon's primary foe.

In the face of horrendous drawbacks, instead of giving up, liver transplantation became an obsession. Starzl became a liver transplantation "addict". He began working excessively long hours, seven days a week, depriving himself of sleep, often reducing it to two hours per day, sacrificing not only his marriage, but also his own health, until his heart began to fail him. He underwent heart surgery several times during his life. This is how the book begins: "The impulse [to record these memoirs] had become more insistent after I underwent two operations on my heart" (p. ix). In 1962, by the time he had reached the age of 36, life had become "a round-the-clock nightmare":

> I operated early in the morning, beginning at 6:00 or 6:30 A.M., arrived at the experimental laboratory by 9:00 or 10:00 in the morning. Work there lasted long past dinner time so that evening rounds or examination of patients to be operated on the following day put off returning home even more. Knowing fatigue was my enemy, I learned to fall asleep in strange places. It was like self-hypnosis. I left home at 4:00 A.M, drove 100 or more miles a day and on lucky days returned home in time to hear the Star-Spangled Banner at 2 A.M. after the last television movie finished. (p. 80/1)

During a self-imposed moratorium on liver transplantation, Starzl temporarily focussed on kidney transplantation (as a surrogate) for some years. The use of captive donors (prisoners), primates (chimpanzees) and reimbursed living donors was considered, but light at the end of the tunnel was eventually offered by two events: the brain-death criterion (allowing for the procurement of organs from bodies that were technically still alive) and the discovery of cyclosporine (to suppress rejection). Meanwhile, the memoirs abound with stories of heroism and self-sacrifice by both patients and physicians. For example, Starzl tells the story of two young colleagues who, chronically fatigued, fell asleep at the wheel, crashing their car in a mountain pass. Although one of them miraculously survived, the other person died, whereupon his liver and kidneys were transplanted (p. 171).

For a long time, the tension between "the perfect world of liver transplantation" as it was imagined, and the "world as it really was" seemed insurmountable (p. 191). Resistance against liver transplantation was not only offered by the bodies of recipients, however, but also by growing numbers of physicians, scientists, politicians, journalists, insurance companies and others. In was only in the 1980s that Starzl managed to decide the "liver wars" (243 ff.) in his favour, with the help of a cohort of fresh young recruits (p. 257), adding more heroic stories (such as the one about an airplane that almost crashed in Nova Scotia, while passenger Starzl, on his way to remove a donor liver, continued to work stoically on an article that was overdue, p. 262/3).

At a certain point, the string nonetheless "broke". Completely exhausted after a 24-hour liver operation, he received an emergency call from another hospital, jumped into a helicopter, and arrived just in time to save the life of a juvenile patient. From that day onwards, however, although electrocardiograms continued to seem normal for some time, he sensed "a strange presence" inside his chest (p. 311). Finally, in 1990, during his first vacation in seven years, a mysterious fatigue came over him. Back in office, he suddenly found himself paralysed on the floor "like a statue". After an hour or so, he recovered and managed to work himself through a pile of mail for another 12 hours before returning home. He had finally become a patient himself, with an angina pectoris-like heart condition, although he decided to chair the biennial meeting of the Transplantation Society in San Francisco before allowing himself to be taken into the operation room. From a Lacanian perspective the question is: what is it that transforms a promising physician into an obsessive workaholic? How did transplantation medicine (as an exemplification of *university discourse*) become trapped in the *matheme of desire* ($\$ \Diamond a$), so that Starzl (as transplantation expert: S_2) became an addict and a patient: a divided and tormented subject ($\$$)?

Basically, the answer is given by Starzl himself. Throughout his career, he suffered from a remarkable symptom, a strange anxiety, which he already noticed in 1958, very early in his career, namely an anxiety to operate—quite remarkable for a hyperactive surgeon with such a career path:

> I harboured anxieties which I was unable to discuss openly until more than three decades later, after I had stopped operating. I had an intense fear of failing the patients who had placed their health or life in my hands... the

anxieties grew worse. Even for simple operations. I would go to the operating room sick with apprehension, almost unable to function until the case began. Later in life, when I told close friends that I did not like to operate, they did not believe me or thought I was joking. (p. 59)

Apparently, his decision to become fixated on the liver, as a tremendous surgical *challenge*, was a case of over-compensation, "subconsciously" chosen to overcome the chronic phobia that threatened to hamper his budding surgical career. If such an operation failed, who would blame him? And if he would be able to successfully transplant a liver, what would be left to fear? Thus, surgeon Starzl fell prey to the formula $\$ \lozenge a$. The only way to compensate the recipients of liver transplants (whom he seemed to be constantly failing) was to work himself into exhaustion, so that he became a patient himself, finally finding the time to recount the story of his life. The liver as his object *a* remained beyond his grasp. Normalcy could never be restored. The object *a* proved unable to domesticate. From the point of view of bodily integrity, every liver transplant, even a successful one, remains a failure, as the implanted organ remains an extimate object of concern for life.

REFERENCE

Starzl, T. 1992/2003. *The Puzzle People. Memoirs of a Transplant Surgeon.* Pittsburgh/London: University of Pittsburgh Press.

CHAPTER 13

The Transplant Organ As an Extimate Object

Abstract In the case of a faltering organ, a particular kind of gap or void emerges, somewhere in the intimacy of our body, an emptiness which Lacan refers to as a vacuole. Medical diagnostic equipment may point out that something is indeed absent or dysfunctional inside. Special contrivances are developed to compensate these deficiencies, turning humans into "prosthetic gods", as Freud phrased it. Today, however, transplantation medicine entails the promise that we may bypass such ersatz solutions to focus directly on the thing (the replaceable organ) itself. The one thing that would allow us to put an end to our chronic deficiencies, making us whole again (the transplantable organ), is not simply available in the outside world, however, in the sense of ready-at-hand. It can only become available as an artefact procured and produced by transplantation medicine. The thing on which our life and well-being (as craving subjects) depends, may still be hidden inside the intimacy of the other's body (either living or brain-dead). Partial objects (such as kidneys) suddenly stand out from the rest of the body. They become detachable from the body as a whole.

Keywords Lacanian psychoanalysis • Extimacy • Replacement
• The uncanny • Brain death • Insatiable organ demand • Idealisation

From a Lacanian perspective, as we have seen, objects of desire convey a promise: to fill the void or gap we experience as craving subjects. For a craving, tormented subject ($) they function as replacements or substi-

© The Author(s) 2019
H. A. E. Zwart, *Purloined Organs*,
https://doi.org/10.1007/978-3-030-05354-3_13

tutes for the lost (or even impossible) "object *a*" as we have seen. The dynamics of human desire are captured by the matheme of desire ($ \$ \lozenge a $) where "*a*" functions not only as the *target* but also as the *cause* of desire. The alluring but inexorable object fuels the awareness of what we lack.

This sense of lack, this gap, can be associated with specific body parts: with faltering organs of various kinds. Building on Freud's conviction that human sexuality is seriously disabled (1930/1948), Lacan's prototype of the unreliable, inexorable object of desire is the *phallic object* (φ), an organ which purportedly is there to serve us but often fails us.[1] According to Lacan, in the aftermath of the oedipal trauma, human sexuality suffers from deficiency and impotence (−φ). In contrast to (other) animals, human beings are *Mängelwesen*, lacking something which (other) animals have, a natural attunement or pre-established harmony between organ and object, body and environment, desire and gratification. Erotic desire builds on the belief that this unreliable item (φ) may actually show up elsewhere. The Other may be seen as someone who *has* the very thing we ourselves are deprived of, for instance, in the case of fetishism: the erotic belief that the (female) Other (A) is secretly in possession of the phallic object of desire (*a*). Rather than as a source of disappointment and frustration (Ⱥ), the Other (A) suddenly emerges as a being in possession of the very thing we seek (Ⱥ + *a* = A). Health problems connected to hearts or kidneys may be seen in a similar manner, as displacements of the original experience of insufficiency associated with the object *a*, a questionable entity from the very outset. It also explains the element of perversion at work in university discourse in general, but particularly in Starzl's obsession with the human liver.

Lacan endorses Marx's analysis of commodity fetishism as outlined above. The alluring aura of the commodity on display builds on the conviction that this particular article may provide us with the very thing we (unconsciously) lack, so that the enticing object, should it fall into our hands, would change the tonality of our whole existence, making us whole again. Yet, the fetish is not the thing itself, but rather a (deceptive) substitute, and therefore bound to frustrate us even more. What would happen if the partial organ *itself* would suddenly be for sale, and would suddenly be transformed into a market commodity? Would our lack finally be healed, our moment of jouissance finally arrive?

---

[1] Cf. the opening lines of *Le Devin du Village*, the opera composed by Jean-Jacques Rousseau: "J'ai perdu tout mon bonheur / J'ai perdu mon serviteur".

These issues are explicitly discussed by Lacan (1968–1969/2006) as we have seen. In the case of a faltering organ, a particular kind of gap or void emerges, somewhere in the intimacy of our body, an emptiness which he refers to as a "vacuole" (p. 232). Medical diagnostic equipment may point out that something is indeed absent or dysfunctional inside. Something is not there, or fails to be in place, or refuses to function properly. Perhaps the disablement is caused by something which should *not* be there, a (removable?) tumorous swelling, an insalubrious partial object?

Before the advent of transplantation medicine, suffering individuals counteracted their deficits with the help of particular EAT ME/DRINK ME consumables (pharmaceuticals) or special contrivances (eventually turning themselves into a "prosthetic god", Freud 1930/1948), but transplantation medicine now entails the promise that we may bypass such ersatz solutions to focus directly on the thing (the replaceable organ) itself. The one thing that would allow us to put an end to our chronic deficiencies, making us whole again, namely the transplantable organ, is not simply available in the outside world, however, in the sense of ready-at-hand. It can only be available as an artefact procured and produced by transplantation medicine. The thing on which our life and well-being (as craving subjects) depends, may still be hidden inside the intimacy of the Other's body (either living or brain-dead). It remains something utterly beyond our grasp as individuals; in Lacanian terminology, it remains something utterly "real". And yet, due to transplantation medicine, this *thing* may now be brought out into the open, may be harvested, brought to the surface, commoditised and revealed as object *a*. The impossible, ungraspable object may suddenly be there, offered to us by high-tech surgery. In the light of this technology-based possibility, other people's organs become a focus of attention, as tantalising objects of desire ($ ◊ *a*). Something which *seemed* firmly embedded within another person's body, becomes detachable and transferable, and this unleashes the desire of craving subjects ($). There finally seems to be an object (*a*) which can possibly make them enjoy life again.

Due to transplantation medicine, certain partial objects (such as kidneys) suddenly *stand out* from the rest of the body; they become detachable, as it were, from the body as a whole. To paraphrase Saint Paul (1 Corinthians 12:15–16), they seem to step out from the body, saying: "I am no longer part of this body". This experience concurs with insights gained in psychoanalysis, where it notably applies to appendix-like body parts such as penises, nipples and breasts (or even teeth: in "typical dreams" about losing one or all of one's teeth for instance). By virtue of their bulging, appendix-like shape, these partial organs raise the (unsettling) suspicion that, apparently, certain segments of human bodies (even highly valued ones) can be absent (the absence of breasts in males, of penises in females), and may be detached or replaced, by oral or phallic artefacts for instance, such as dildos or comforters.

Since the 1950s, transplantation medicine has reinforced and amplified this idea, Lacan argues, introducing a new set of detachable organs into the dynamics of desire. As a result, the Thomistic idea (once dominant) of the body as an inviolable whole became increasingly questionable and recessive. The very fact that organs can be procured, even from living donors, so that faltering originals can be replaced, confirms the idea that the body is *not* an indivisible unity. Integrity is *not* a characteristic of the real body, but rather a feature which pertains to the "imaginary", that is, the idealised, illusory, aestheticised *ideal* body (Lacan 1968–1969/2006, p. 270).

In short, from a Lacanian perspective, transplantation medicine is a technological development with important ontological repercussions. It entails an ontological revelation, an opening-up of the human body to fragmentation. Various organs and body parts may be taken out and replaced by partial objects of desire, procurable from others. For a craving subject, a transplant organ becomes an extremely valuable thing, carrying the promise of survival and jouissance (in technocratic language: "quality of life"). Yet, these biomedical promises incarnated in transplant organs are bound to entail frustrations of their own. A transplant organ is a *pharmakon*, both beneficial and poisonous, and every techno-scientific solution creates new challenge and problems. Rejection and life-long dependence on immunosuppressant drugs are symptomatic of the fact that the fit between the *real* body of the recipient and the transplanted, embedded organ (however alluring) will remain sub-optimal. The implanted organ remains, as Lacan aptly phrases it, an "extimate" object (1968–1969/2006): a paradoxical entity, both internal and external, both intimate and foreign, both life-saving and alienating, or even toxic—an item of concern and anxiety for years to come as we have seen. Even if the new organ appears to function well, it remains tainted by otherness, both biologically (upsetting the body's immune system) and figuratively (as an organ which at one time belonged to someone else and still carries this other person's genetic signature).

On 26 June 1969, Lacan (1968–1969/2006) explicitly discusses recent developments in transplantation medicine. Organ transplants are explicitly framed as "objects a". An object *a*, Lacan argues, is first and foremost a transferable, detachable, alienable object (objet cessible, p. 362). This applies, for example, to the breast during the oral stage. Initially, young children experience the breast/nipple as part of themselves: a partial organ belonging to their own body while being nourished. The child is literally (physically) "attached" to it. That the breast/nipple can be removed at all, gives rise to an experience of profound surprise on the part of the neonate. In other words, initially, the breast is not regarded by the new-born infant as an "object" at all.

A quintessential feature of the object *a* is its apparent replaceability. The breast of a doe may replace the mother's breast: a major concern for romanticist Jean-Jacques Rousseau, who vehemently argued that mothers should breast-feed their own offspring. But a breast may also be replaced by comforters, available as commodities in supermarkets. Thus, techno-logically reproducible artefacts become stand-ins for natural objects, so that objects of desire seemingly become replaceable by commodities of all sorts. This is already implied by the fact that these partial objects (breast, penis, hand, eye, etc.) tend to have the form of a detachable, replaceable body part (p. 363), shaped like an appendix, a bulging extension.

All these artificial replacements (comforters, etc.) still mimic the natural organ: they are instances of "Anlehnung". A further step is taken, a further technological "revelation" occurs (Lacan 1968–1969/2006, p. 363) when organs *as such* become replaceable. Now, the transferable, replace-able nature of the object *a* (the thing that purports to save someone's life) is emphasised even more emphatically, due to organ transplantation. Developments in this area are so breath-taking and remarkable, Lacan argues, that we may well wonder whether certain moral "limits" are to be set (p. 363). Indeed, transplantation medicine is an ontological gold mine, a resource of astonishing possibilities. It is even possible, Lacan explains, to artificially keep human bodies in a brain-dead state, mid-way between life and death. Their organs and tissues remain alive, although their cere-bral functions are irreversibly destroyed. Would it be allowed to harvest organs from such an undead body, turning it into a resource, ready-at-hand? This possibility invokes the question whether human beings are merely their bodies (p. 364). Indeed, the possibility of organ procurement from brain-dead patients even revivifies the (allegedly outdated) question concerning the existence of a human soul. On the other hand, Lacan argues, taking a more anticipatory turn, one may argue that these technical developments actually prepare the ground for what may be seen as the hypermodern version of the resurrected body, as envisioned by Christianity, but now sublated by modern techno-science: the quasi-immortal body of regenerative medicine.

Lacan also refers to Freud who, in his essay on "The uncanny" (*das Unheimliche*, 1919/1947), discusses E.T.A. Hoffmann's story *The Sandman*, about Olimpia's replaceable eyes, which apparently can be removed from and reinserted into their sockets, bringing her to life as it were, and which are therefore both fascinating and deterring, both alluring and disconcerting. As transferrable objects *a* (representing the *optic* object *a*), they exemplify the uncanny par excellence. Other technologies may also produce replicas, Lacan argues, such as recordings (reproducing the human voice) or pictures and video-tapes (capturing the human gaze). Indeed, a plethora of techniques have become available for boosting the transferability and storability of objects of desire, making their presence ubiquitous in contemporary Western societies. Public spaces are *pervaded* by (representations of) the faces, gazes, voices and (nude) body parts of others, and this includes, one could argue, advertisements summoning reluctant citizens to become organ donors, ostensibly exhibiting the faces, voices and bodies of craving recipients *before* implantation, in sharp contrast with pictures of exuberantly happy and healthy recipients *after* the operation, to amplify the message.

Pro-donation propaganda addresses audience on three levels. First of all, via the *symbolic*, providing quantitative data of moribund patients on waiting lists, appealing to us to sign up as potential organ donors. But they also address us by way of the *imaginary*: via the exaggeratingly healthy bodies and faces of transplantation survivors, on billboards and in magazines. Finally, there is the register of the *real*: the obscene view of bodies being operated upon, whose sternum has just been split or whose peritoneum has just been slit open, allowing us to peer into the bloody mess inside, invoking mixtures of curiosity and repulsion. It would be naïve to think, however, that the demand for organs can be met if only the number of available donor organs would increase. Quite the contrary: to the extent that transplantation medicine becomes successful, and the number of procurable organs increases, the demand for organs will continue to increase as well. For Lacan, organ hunger will prove insatiable in the end.

References

Freud, S. 1919/1947. Das Unheimliche. In *Gesammelte Werke XII*, 227–268. London: Imago.

———. 1930/1948. Das Unbehagen in der Kultur. In *Gesammelte Werke XIV*, 419–513. London: Imago.

Lacan, J. 1968–1969/2006. *Le Séminaire de Jacques Lacan XVI: D'un Autre à l'autre*. Paris: Éditions du Seuil.

CHAPTER 14

Separation and Desire

Abstract Another Lacanian concept relevant for coming to terms with transplantation medicine is the complex of separation (from the mother's body). As foetuses, humans nest as parasites inside the motherly womb, where all vital needs are lavishly met. The birth trauma is a choking experience, however, and although breast-feeding is meant to uphold a certain level of proximity and intimacy, new experiences of separation and frustration await the new-born child. The idea of the missing part first and foremost applies to the placenta. What makes technological substitutes alluring is their promise to fill up the emptiness resulting from the loss. The disavowal of the irreversible nature of the loss gives rise to a production line of substitutes, purporting to fill the gap. Craving subjects may become fixated on a particular object in an obsessive manner, resulting in a radical narrowing of focus, as Žižek phrases it. The partial object becomes a fetish: something which purports to suture the missing part. Against this backdrop, the benevolent/toxic organ implant surfaces as a paragon object of desire.

Keywords Vulnerability • Aristophanes • Birth trauma • Discontent • Artefacts • Anatomy • Displacement

From a Lacanian perspective, humans emerge not as entities who *have* something which (other) animals *lack* (rationality, self-consciousness, big brains, a soul, etc.), but rather as beings who *lack* something which (other)

© The Author(s) 2019   69
H. A. E. Zwart, *Purloined Organs*,
https://doi.org/10.1007/978-3-030-05354-3_14

animals *have* (a natural attunement or correspondence between instinct and *Umwelt*, between bodily needs and habitat; Zwart 2014, 2016, 2017). Humans are born prematurely into this world, unable to either walk or talk. Even as adults, they cannot sleep without blankets nor trust their instincts. Although equipped with freely moveable hands, much of their time is spent on artificial crutches known as furniture (chairs, beds, etc.; Žižek 2010, p. 87). Humans are unhappy, stunted creatures from the very outset: divided, craving and tormented subjects (in Lacanian algebra: $), suffering from a chronic misfit between what they desire and what is expected of them. And rather than solve our problems, technology (once unleashed) will reveal and amplify this radical imbalance, this primal discord at the very core of human existence (Žižek 2004/2012, p. 109).

In other words, Lacanian psychoanalysis basically concurs with the view of Arnold Gehlen and others of humans as *deficient* beings or *Mängelwesen* (Gehlen 1940/1962) whose "organ inferiority" (Adler 1927/2009) becomes compensated by culture, language and contrivances: by the symbolic order, providing a life-line, a protective shelter against the threatening Real—technology as "vulnerability coping" (Coeckelbergh 2015). But compensations inevitably become sources of malaise in their own right, because of culture's inherent tendency to become excessive, giving rise to overcompensation, so that rather than serving us, the techno-symbolic order haunts us and preys on us (Zwart 2016, 2017). We are not only fundamentally dependent upon but also pervaded by biomedical techno-science. From a Lacanian perspective, biomedical techno-science is an imperious mechanism, cleaving and infecting subjects, relentlessly colonising their world.

For Lacan, seeing ourselves as autonomous agents (who merely *use* certain artefacts to realise their goals) is as misguided as seeing ourselves as beautiful souls (who find themselves besieged by a relentlessly advancing technological culture). Rather, we are chronically divided subjects from the very start, craving for something (e.g. a missing object) which seems irrevocably lost. This object loss builds on primordial experiences of separation from parts of ourselves that we have been deprived of (Lacan 1966–1967, 842 ff.), resulting in a chronic sense of gap, invaded by desire and sutured by technology. The classical (albeit farcical) description of this primordial separation experience is Aristophanes' famous myth about hominid beings who (at the start of the humanisation process) were cleft in two, as recorded in Plato's *Symposium* (Plato 1996; cf. Lacan 1938/2001), giving rise to a desperate yearning for the lost complement, as a basic thrust of culture.

This dialectic already surfaces in one of Lacan's earlier texts entitled *Familial Complexes in the Formation of the Individual* (Lacan 1938/2001), where he discusses the complex of separation (from the mother's body). As foetuses, Lacan argues, humans nest as parasites inside the motherly womb, where all vital needs are lavishly met (Lacan 1938/2001, p. 30, cf. 1966–1967, p. 848). Separation (i.e. the birth trauma) is a choking experience and although breast-feeding is meant to uphold a certain level of proximity and intimacy, new experiences of separation and frustration await the new-born child. These may give rise to various symptoms later in life, such as alcoholism, anorexia, or other enacted refusals of the questionable replacements offered as substitutes for the irretrievably lost object: the placenta, the primordial nipple or breast, and so forth—in Lacanian algebra, the object *a*. The persevering refusal of this inevitable separation (from a prototypically "lost object") fuels repetitive efforts to artificially restore parasitic, nourishing relationships later in life, revolving around the scar or void that was left behind, outlining the lost object's haunting image.[1]

Thus, during extra-uterine existence, humans frantically aim to establish living conditions which mimic the lost original position as convincingly as possible.[2] And it is here that culture and technology step in, whose basic objective is to restore (to a certain extent) the vanished protective sphere. Yet, as Freud (1930/1948) already argued in *Civilisation and its Discontents*, this basic programme of culture and technology is bound to fall short, because aside from solving certain problems, techno-scientific artefacts will inevitably introduce a host of new complications as well. Because we easily become dependent on these substitutes, they become sources of discontent in their own right, while human existence continues to be marked by frustration, frantic longing and chronic desire.

This situation is captured by Lacan's matheme of desire as we have seen ($ \$ \lozenge a $), where $\$$ (barred S) represents the split (tormented, craving)

---

[1] Here again, Lacan refers to the severed breasts of Saint Agatha (albeit using Giovanni Batista Tiepolo's version on this occasion) to emphasise that the irretrievably lost object can only be envisioned at the very moment of its disappearance, as a transient snapshot, such as in the case of falling stars at night, or elementary particles in cloud chambers, or a paralysing, captivating glance, spotted briefly and in passing.

[2] This idea was elaborated by Peter Sloterdijk (1998, 487 ff.), both building on and criticising Lacan (Sloterdijk and Heinrichs 2001, 12 ff.).

subject and *a* the lost, impossible, inexorable object (the object-cause of human desire); while the diamond (lozenge, *poinçon*) in the middle can be read as an arrow pointing in both directions, so that desire, besides functioning as a vector oriented towards the missing object's coordinates, may also be aroused by particular items which present themselves as alluring substitutes, making us aware of what we lack and conveying the promise that the script of our core phantasy can still be realised.

The idea of the missing part (the absent *partial object*) first and foremost applies to the placenta, as we have seen: our primordial life-saving, organic extension symbolising the lost object *a* in a rather profound way (Lacan 1964/1973, p. 221). In his seminar on anxiety, Lacan argues that the first primordial trauma is indeed the experience of being born (Lacan 1962–1963/2004, p. 362): the exodus from the womb, the experience of being slit from the placenta, and the separation anxiety resulting from this. From the new-born's perspective, the motherly breast emerges as a kind of externalised placenta, loosely attached to the maternal body as a soothing remainder: something which actually seems to belong to the body of the child, something to which he or she seems entitled (Lacan 1966–1967, p. 256).

Thus, during the nursing stage, young children still experience themselves as fused, more or less, with the mother's body. They do not yet perceive themselves as fully separate entities and do not yet see the breast as an "object", but rather as something which somehow continues to belong to their own corporeal self. During breast feeding, the breast and nipple stand out as temporary extensions whose surface smoothly folds itself to the oral mucous membrane. But this experience of fusion is illusory and untenable. The separation experience becomes repetitive, giving rise to additional frustrations. Replacement of the organic object (i.e. the mother's breast) soon becomes an option, and the soothing function may be transferred to a doe, for instance,[3] or to artificial comforters, feeding bottles and so on. This is where technology enters the scene. The organic original becomes a replaceable, transferrable (cessible) object (1962–1963/2004, p. 363)—replaceable by substitutes (plastic or otherwise) purporting to mimic it, in function as well as in shape.[4] Technology

---

[3] At one time a widespread practice to which Jean-Jacques Rousseau (as a true Romantic) vehemently objected, in one of the first scholarly publications devoted to this subject.

[4] Lacan repeatedly refers to Donald Winnicott who sees childhood toys and dolls (such as teddy bears) as transitional objects (both external and intimate, both real and illusory) which

thus produces a host of potential substitutes: technologically reproducible partial objects, alluring but deceptive replacements of the real (lost) thing. These substitutes cannot really gratify desire, however, and the awareness of the painful, insatiable loss will continue to torment us.

For Lacan, building on Freud, another instance of a faltering object, unleashing the dynamics of human desire, is the phallus. Unlike Freud, Lacan emphasises that it does not refer to the (physical, visible, organic) penis (Verhaeghe 2001, p. 10), but rather to the phallus as a *symbolic* item, functioning as an irretrievably lost (and only partially replaceable) spectral thing (whose absence is denoted as: $-\varphi$). The phallic object a is not something we may or may not "have", ready at hand, but rather something whose presence and performance remain highly precarious: something anatomical only in the *etymological* sense of the term (where ἀνα-τομία refers to bodily items that can be or have been cut away). As Žižek phrases it, notwithstanding its obstinacy, the phallic object a has no positive ontological consistency (Žižek 2010, p. 69), so that we are chronically in need of stand-ins. Consider, for instance, the stereotypical gun in Western movies, or the enchanted sword in early medieval or Samurai tales, or Uma Thurman's katana (skilfully employed in *Kill Bill* movies to take revenge upon her perpetrators by chopping off arms and legs and tearing out eyes). For Lacan, (the lack of) the phallic object ($-\varphi$) basically refers to a vacancy at the core of human existence, amounting to the inability of individuals to overcome their impasses and achieve their goals, that is, to satisfy the desires of others as well as of themselves. Various objects (artificial replacements) purport to suture this void (Ragland 1995, p. 189) and biomedicine provides us with a plethora of questionable compensations to counteract the chronic malaise (in Lacanian algebra: $a/-\varphi$). In other words, the function of technology is not primarily to satisfy bodily (biological) needs, but rather to produce alluring semblances, enticing objects of desire, arousing in us a craving that goes beyond the mere satisfaction of physiological urges, promising singular forms of *jouissance* which are currently denied to us. Although the desirable object (the transplantable organ) may easily be mistaken for the thing itself, it is actually a lure, invested with libido and fetishised by desire.

---

may soothe and facilitate the inevitable destruction of the symbiotic mother-child relationship by temporarily replacing the object a. A fetish, Lacan adds, is basically a frozen transitory object for adults (Lacan 1967–1968, pp. 35–36, 1956–1957/1994, pp. 34–35).

The common factor of various (oral, anal or phallic) replacements is that they are connected with experiences of loss as well as with bodily orifices, pointing out the gaps (Verhaeghe 2001). Rather than using natural orifices, however, organ implantation creates an artificial opening or slit, a neo-mouth, where the procured organ is to be inserted, leaving a scar. Besides the lost objects discussed so far, moreover, Lacan adds two additional items to the set, namely the scopic object a (the gaze of the Other, associated with the eye as an organ and the pupil as an orifice) and the auditory object a (the voice of the Other, associated with the ear as an organ and the auditory channel as an orifice).[5] The missing item $(-\varphi)$ becomes a vector of desire, giving rise to a relentless quest for the alluring entity that technological substitutes purport to mimic. Lacan connects this with the Freudian mechanism of displacement (*Verschiebung*) and with the linguistic concept of metonymy: the tendency of desire to continuously shift its target, to remain dissatisfied, to keep craving for "something else"—resulting in endless deferral, so that the insatiable quest for the lost object becomes an interminable adventure.

What makes technological substitutes alluring is their promise to fill up the emptiness resulting from the loss $(a/-\varphi)$. The disavowal of the inexorable nature of the loss gives rise to an interminable process of multiplication, a production line of substitutes, purporting to fill the gap (Žižek 2006/2009, p. 61). Biomedical options for replacement will continue to become available in the future, claiming to mimic the lost original as closely as possible. In accordance with the matheme of desire ($\$ \lozenge a$), subjects will cling to these options, fuelled by the unconscious conviction that the phantasmatic object may somehow still exist. Subjects may become fixated on a singular object in an obsessive manner, so that all daily activities begin to circulate around it, resulting in a radical narrowing of focus (Žižek 2004/2012, p. 127). The partial object becomes a fetish: something which purports to 'suture' the missing part $(a/-\varphi)$. Against this backdrop, the benevolent/toxic organ implant, which may or may not become available in time, surfaces as a paragon object of desire.

---

[5] Building on Aristophanes' parable in *Symposium*, Lacan further explores this experience of profound loss by arguing that it gives rise to a "lamella", an ultra-thin surface (Lacan 1966–1967, p. 847; Lacan 1964/1973, p. 222), a flexible remainder of the traumatic cut, a two-dimensional, fictitious "organ", attaching itself (as a highly sensitive film) to corporeal orifices (mouth, anus, the inner mucosa of vagina or penis, etc.), thereby creating erogenous zones, instilling in human individuals a yearning for something to which they somehow seem entitled and which they apparently cannot do without.

References

Adler, A. 1927/2009. *Menschenkenntnis*. Frankfurt am Main: Fischer.

Coeckelbergh, M. 2015. The Art of Living with ICTs: The Ethics–Aesthetics of Vulnerability Coping and Its Implications for Understanding and Evaluating ICT Cultures. *Foundations of Science* 22 (2): 339–348.

Freud, S. 1930/1948. Das Unbehagen in der Kultur. In *Gesammelte Werke XIV*, 419–513. London: Imago.

Gehlen, A. 1940/1962. *Der Mensch. Seine Natur und seine Stellung in der Welt*. Frankfurt: Athenäum.

Lacan, J. 1938/2001. Les complexes familiaux dans la formation de l'individu: Essai d'analyse d'une fonction en psychologie. In *Autres Écrits*, 23–84. Paris: Éditions du Seuil.

———. 1956–1957/1994. *Le Séminaire de Jacques Lacan IV: La relation d'objet et les structures freudiennes*. Paris: Éditions du Seuil.

———. 1962–1963/2004. *Le Séminaire de Jacques Lacan X: L'Angoisse*. Paris: Éditions du Seuil.

———. 1964/1973. *Le séminaire de Jacques Lacan XI: Les quatre concepts fondamentaux de la psychanalyse*. Paris: Éditions du Seuil.

———. 1966–1967. *Le séminaire XIV: Logique du fantasme* (unpublished). http://staferla.free.fr/.

———. 1967–1968. *Le Séminaire de Jacques Lacan XV: L'acte de la psychanalyse* (unpublished). http://staferla.free.fr/.

Plato. 1925/1996. *Lysis, Symposium, Gorgias*. Loeb ed. Cambridge: Harvard University Press.

Ragland, E. 1995. The Relation Between the Voice and the Gaze. In *Reading Seminar XI: Lacan's Four Fundamental Concepts of Psychoanalysis*, ed. Richard Feldstein, Bruce Fink, and Maire Jaanus, 187–203. Albany: State University of New York Press.

Sloterdijk, P. 1998. *Sphären I: Blasen*. Frankfurt: Suhrkamp.

Sloterdijk, P., and H.-J. Heinrichs. 2001. *Die Sonne und der Tod: Dialogische Untersuchungen*. Frankfurt: Suhrkamp.

Verhaeghe, P. 2001. *Beyond Gender: From Subject to Drive*. New York: Other Press.

Žižek, S. 2004/2012. *Organs Without Bodies: On Deleuze and Consequences*. London/New York: Routledge.

———. 2006/2009. *The Parallax View*. Cambridge/London: The MIT Press

———. 2010. *Living in the End Times*. London/New York: Verso.

Zwart, H. 2014. The Donor Organ as an 'Object A': A Lacanian Perspective on Organ Donation and Transplantation Medicine. *Medicine, Health Care & Philosophy: A European Journal* 17 (4): 559–571. https://doi.org/10.1007/s11019-014-9553-1.

————. 2016. Transplantation Medicine, Organ Theft Cinema and Bodily Integrity. *Subjectivity* 9 (2): 151–180. https://doi.org/10.1057/sub.2016.1.

————. 2017. Extimate' Technologies and Techno-Cultural Discontent: A Lacanian Analysis of Pervasive Gadgets. *Techné: Research in Philosophy and Technology* 21 (1): 24–54. https://doi.org/10.5840/techne2017456.

CHAPTER 15

Bios and Techne

Abstract Transplants and implants not only promise to suture the gap, but also reveal something which has been there from the very outset. Extimacy is not a recent by-product of biomedical techno-science, but an endogenous dimension of human embodiment as such. Transplantation medicine reveals the extent to which extimacy (notably the intimate-detachable status of particular organs such as testicles and breasts) constitutes a basic dimension of embodied existence.

Keywords Vacuole • Extimacy • Implants • Narcissistic offence • Partial objects • Working-through

Biomedical interventions aim to restore the functionality of the human organism, targeting or even replacing the dysfunctional body part. Lacan explicitly discusses transplantation medicine, as we have seen (Lacan 1968–1969/2006, p. 363), stressing that developments in this area move forward very quickly and will continue to surprise us, such as the harvesting of organs from brain-dead persons, artificially kept alive for no other purpose (p. 364). We have outlined how, in the case of a faltering organ, an emptiness emerges in the intimacy of the body, a "vacuole" (1968–1969/2006, p. 224, p. 232), once occupied by the now dysfunctional body part ($-\varphi$), so that the vector of desire pushes the craving subject towards the organ implant as a possible life-line: the object a of

© The Author(s) 2019   77
H. A. E. Zwart, *Purloined Organs*,
https://doi.org/10.1007/978-3-030-05354-3_15

transplantation medicine, allegedly suturing the gap $(a/-\varphi)$. The implant will prove a highly precarious solution, however, as the new organ is bound to become an issue of concern in its own right, a candidate for future replacements. Such replacements constitute intimate/alienating artefacts, both embedded and foreign, both life-saving and intrusive. This ambiguity is captured by the concept of extimacy, as we have seen, conjoining the notion of intimacy with that of radical exteriority (Lacan 1968–1969/2006, p. 224, p. 249), allowing us to stipulate the ambiguous position of the "extimate object a" (p. 249) and its substitutes.

There is the possibility of course that the extimate object a of a future transplantation medicine will no longer be something organic, but rather an implantable gadget, something which *obliterates* the organic thing, containing a chip or a small computer (Zwart 2017). Such implants have already begun to enter our life-worlds and bodies in the form of biochips, neuro-implants, artificial heart valves and artificial kidneys, so that organic emptiness will be sutured by smart, implantable and biocompatible gadgets $(a/-\varphi)$. Such extimate objects entail a shift of focus from the external environment to the increased manipulability of the human organism as such. Technologically reproducible implants claim to assist us in our frantic efforts to enjoy life, but, at the same time, they are nonetheless likely to become an object of intense concern: is the gadget still functioning properly? Should the extimate object falter, new intrusions are doubtlessly awaiting us. Implants expose recipients to permanent monitoring and surveillance, to the voice and gaze of the Big Other (Φ) on whom they increasingly come to depend. Extimate implants act as seductive substitutes, purporting to replace the irretrievably lost object with a more sophisticated version $(a/-\varphi)$. At the same time, they focus on the craving human subject $(\$)$ directly and transform the recipient's body into an object of control with the help of computerised devices. Thus, transplantation medicine is part of the inward turn of technology. The traditional technological situation involves an organ which is supplemented by an instrument (ὄργανον in Greek) so as to make the outside world more manageable and survival-friendly, although this supplement often profoundly affects the human body and its organs in return, so that a process of coevolution is unleashed: a complex interplay of the organic and the mechanic, of human embodiment and technology. In other words, while humans are reshaping (humanising) the outside world, they also re-sculpt (domesticated) themselves as well, so that we are not only the product of a natural, but also of techno-cultural evolution. Our tools and contrivances allow us to appear as subjects who are, to a significant extent, self-made (Stiegler 2010; Zwart 2009; Lemmens 2015). Currently, we are becoming the target of self-reengineering much more directly, via implants and gadgets which invade us rather than extend us. In many cases, these entities will remain erratic implants, however, due to their failure to become really embedded in the body as a whole (Žižek 2006/2009, pp. 122–123, 2004/2012, p. 156), but the alternative scenario, namely that some of them become embedded quite smoothly, efficiently, and intimately, must be taken into account as well.

Psychoanalytically speaking it would be naïve to think that transplantation medicine will primarily allow us to overcome our corporeal shortcomings. Implants will prove beneficial and toxic at the same time, and it is their inherent toxicity which tends to be obfuscated by proclamations of the coming of a bright and happy future: the regeneratable body. Moreover, to add another dialectical twist, transplants and implants may reveal or emphasise something which has been there from the very outset, namely extimacy *not* as a recent by-product of biomedical techno-science, but as an endogenous dimension of human embodiment as such (Zwart 2017). Human bodies are inherently pervaded by intrusive entities in a very profound way: beneficial and toxic at the same time, for what applies to biomedical implants already applies to our natural organs as well. Extimate implants undermine a reassuring, but imaginary view of the human body as something which once existed in a natural, unviolated state, thereby revealing an unsettling truth. Rather than unleashing a completely new situation (without precedent in the history of evolution), transplantation medicine actually reveals the extent to which extimacy constitutes a basic dimension of embodied life itself. The extimacy of partial objects is something Real, obfuscated perhaps by various fictitious images of the body's wholeness, integrity and inviolability, but now relentlessly brought out into the open, giving rise to a narcissistic offence, challenging our sense of dignity, individuality and agency.

This already applies to the classic Freudian set of partial objects discussed above. The motherly breast (the oral object *a*) for instance, while providing a life-line to new-born infants, may well become a toxic, metastatic threat to the mothers themselves, an extimate object arousing suspicion, giving rise to practices like regular check-ups or self-monitoring, or even preventive removal, so as to forego cancer (the archetypal organic threat from within). In other words, the ambivalent status of extimacy may already apply to this particular appendix-like organ as such.

As to the faeces (the anal object *a*), it is remarkable how, in recent years, human excrements became a focal point of attention in biomedical research no less than in psychoanalytic practice. Life scientists took to studying the gut microbiome (i.e. the millions of microorganisms, *E. coli* and others, inhabiting our intestines, responsible for our metabolism, functioning as benign intruders, but regarding us merely as their ecosystem) while human stool is now increasingly used as a diagnostic tool (for detecting colon cancer for instance) or as a resource for therapy (via faecal microbiota transplants or faecal bacteriotherapy). In other words, what these developments reveal or confirm is the anal object *a* as something which is both me and not-me, both familiar and repellent, both an item of waste and a gift, both detestable and valuable: a view that has been propagated by psychoanalytic literature from the very outset.

Testicles may be regarded as extimate partial objects in a rather palpable manner and their extimate status is already underscored by their curious anatomical position, both inside and outside the body, drenching male bodies (notably during adolescence, but also later in life) in testosterone, a toxic substance, giving rise to excessive, unquenchable desire. But they may also function as model organs whose *modus operandi* may be mimicked by smart, wearable devices, worn on (or directly under) the skin, ejecting electronic signals or bioactive substances (as biochemical signals) into the human organism, urging tissues and organs to respond more adequately to recorded instances of deprivation or excess (as indicated by precision measurements), or simply to invoke specific moods of states of arousal (implants which function as clean, electronic, post-organic gonads as it were).

The phallus is the extimate "organ without a body" par excellence, as Žižek (2004/2012, p. 78) phrases it, attached to bodies, but without really becoming an organic part, rather "sticking out as an excessive, incoherent supplement". As a detachable, external organ, it is connected with gender in a flexible way, because both erotic literature and psychoanalytic practice inform us that the detachable, transferable phallus plays a key role in a plethora of erotic activities and phantasies, ranging from transvestism via masochism up to fetishism. Recently, it was discovered that role reversal (phallus transference) is not exclusively an ingredient of human eroticism (where it has been practised with the help of dildos etc. since time immemorial). In a Brazilian cave, a research team discovered a case of intromittent sexual organ reversal among insects of the genus Neotrogla (Yoshizawa et al. 2014). While females have a highly elaborate, penis-like structure (a *gynosome*), an intromittent organ in males is lacking. In fact, these polyandrous females are equipped with various organs for grasping and holding reluctant males, coercively gripping their sternum, so as to procure gametes from their sperm storage organ (*spermatheca*) while, during the extended copulation process (40–70 hours), male bodies often become fatally mutilated. In the near future perhaps, as a case of what Freud called *Anlehnung* (literally: "to be modelled after" or "to lean-upon"), sensitive, functional and embedded (organic, bionic or hybrid) implants may be developed such that "active" and "passive" roles (as Freudians once phrased it) may become a matter of choice or mood rather than of anatomical destiny. It is no coincidence perhaps that, precisely now that the "phallic woman" phantasm is becoming technologically plausible, this same scenario also emerges as something already biologically real; although the question remains whether the transfiguration of the phallic object into an implant would indeed subvert and expose or rather reinforce the (traditional) psychoanalytic image of phallic pleasure as a gendered "privilege".

Finally, the availability of retinal and cochlear implants may affect the way we assess and experience our natural eyes and ears, as embedded and sophisticated, but at the same time increasingly replaceable and optimisable contrivances, so that smart implants may allow us to fill the gaps, remove the blind spots, increase resolution, broaden the spectrum of detectable frequencies or equip ourselves with an additional (movable) third eye or ear. The availability of micro-implants may point attention to gaps we hardly realised were there, such as our inability to discern infrared light, only noticeable to us as heat. Once installed, however, the gadget may take on a life of its own. A third eye, for instance, may (willingly or unwillingly) become the incarnation of a perverse, stalking drive.

One could even argue that extimacy goes much further back in the history of life and that mitochondria (as powerhouses of eukaryotic cells) may count as the most primordial version of the extimate intruder. The theory is that they once entered the eukaryotic cell as invading or absorbed bacteria (symbionts), as intimate and organic (biocompatible) "devices" so to speak, making eukaryotic life possible (Lane 2005): the cellular version of the forgotten "other", but now incorporated rather than lost. And electronic precision devices may well single out mitochondria as targets of choice, to address symptoms of depression and fatigue, for instance, by manipulating mitochondrial functioning.

Organ transplants operate on both sides of the matheme of desire ($ ◊ a$) as we have seen: not only by (promising to) produce objects of desire which individuals obsessively may want to *have*, but also by pushing craving subjects into certain modes of *being*. Instead of trying to stop the advance of intrusive technologies (whose partial objects will increasingly claim us), a Lacanian way out would be to endorse an ethos of *working through*. Instead of opting for imaginary scenarios (either by yearning for a pristine past or by leaping into a post-human future), this would entail an active questioning of the unfolding present (Gunkel and Taylor 2014).

In 1969, when Lacan presented his seminar on organ transplantation, organ transplants were still highly exceptional, and often even futuristic events, performed by pioneers (world-famous star surgeons), covered by mass media, presenting options which had not really entered the world of normal existence. For subsequent generations of intellectuals, living and ageing in the twenty-first century, however, this has clearly changed. Transplantation medicine has become a real option, so that French intellectuals are no longer merely *discussing* the ontological violence entailed in it (as Lacan did in 1969) but are actually *experiencing* it. This is exemplified by two highly personal accounts by prominent academics who became organ recipients themselves, namely Jean-Luc Nancy (2000/2010) and Francisco Varela (2001). These memoirs concur, I will argue, with Lacan's prognostics, providing valuable case materials to probe and refine our Lacanian perspective.

REFERENCES

Gunkel, D., and P. Taylor. 2014. *Heidegger and the Media*. Cambridge: Polity.
Lacan, J. 1968–1969/2006. *Le Séminaire de Jacques Lacan XVI: D'un Autre à l'autre*. Paris: Éditions du Seuil.
Lane, N. 2005. *Power, Sex, Suicide: Mitochondria and the Meaning of Life*. Oxford/New York: Oxford University Press.
Lemmens, P. 2015. Social Autonomy and Heteronomy in the Age of ICT: The Digital Pharmakon and the (Dis)Empowerment of the General Intellect. *Foundations of Science* 22 (2): 287–296. https://doi.org/10.1007/s10699-015-9468-1.
Nancy, J.-L. 2000/2010. *L'intrus*. Paris: Galilée.
Stiegler, B. 2010. *Ce qui fait que la vie vaut la peine d'être vécue: de la pharmacologie*. Paris: Flammarion.
Varela, F. 2001. Intimate Distances: Fragments for a Phenomenology of Organ Transplantation. *Journal of Consciousness Studies* 8 (5–7): 259–271.

Yoshizawa, K., R. Ferreira, Y. Kamimura, and C. Lienhard. 2014. Female Penis, Male Vagina, and Their Correlated Evolution in a Cave Insect. *Current Biology* 24: 1–5. https://doi.org/10.1016/j.cub.2014.03.022.

Žižek, S. 2004/2012. *Organs Without Bodies: On Deleuze and Consequences.* London/New York: Routledge.

———. 2006/2009. *The Parallax View.* Cambridge/London: The MIT Press

Zwart, H. 2009. From Utopia to Science: Challenges of Personalised Genomics Information for Health Management and Health Enhancement. *Medicine Studies* 1 (2): 155–166.

———. 2017. Extimate' Technologies and Techno-Cultural Discontent: A Lacanian Analysis of Pervasive Gadgets. *Techné: Research in Philosophy and Technology* 21 (1): 24–54. https://doi.org/10.5840/techne2017456.

CHAPTER 16

Revealing Intrusions/Intruding Revelations

Abstract In *The Intruder*, Jean-Luc Nancy describes his experiences as an organ recipient as a "metaphysical adventure". It was the faltering organ itself which created the awkward sense of emptiness in the intimacy of his body, the void or vacuole within his chest. The dysfunctional organ itself is described as the first intruder, the first uncanny object, while the foreign heart implanted into the body unleashes a whole series of subsequent intrusions. They quickly begin to multiply. A similar account was published by Francisco Varela, who underwent a liver transplant and whose memoirs (*Intimate distances*) thematise intrusion as a core experience. Increasingly, individuals will be faced with circulating body parts, passing from one body to the next, redesigning the landscape of corporeal boundaries.

Keywords Case studies • Phenomenology • First person perspective • Intrusiveness • Extimacy

In his essay *L'Intrus* (*The Intruder*), Jean-Luc Nancy (2000/2010) describes his experiences as an organ recipient as a "metaphysical adventure" (p. 14). It was the faltering organ itself, he points out, which created the awkward sense of "emptiness" in the intimacy of his body, the void within his chest (Lacan's vacuole). Indeed, the dysfunctional organ itself is described as the first intruder, the first alien and uncanny object, while the

© The Author(s) 2019   85
H. A. E. Zwart, *Purloined Organs*,
https://doi.org/10.1007/978-3-030-05354-3_16

heart transplant purported to provide a *restitutio ad integrum*, but that proved not at all to be the case. Rather, implanting a stranger's heart into a body unleashes a whole series of subsequent intrusions. They quickly begin to multiply. Although the wound is sutured, the slit is never completely closed, but rather transformed into a scar, while the surviving body is scanned, monitored and exposed meticulously, becoming embedded in a network of connections, routines, check-ups and interventions. The living body is transformed into an android, a "non-unity", an assemblage (p. 51), a patch-work body (corps bricolé, p. 53). According to Nancy, however, the organ transplant merely reveals that the human body is tainted by foreignness and disintegration from the very outset. As Slatman and Widdershoven phrase it, Nancy's analysis reveals that the human body is *always* characterised by strangeness, that one's "own body" is never fully (experienced as) one's own (2010, p. 76). This concurs with Lacan's dictum that human beings experience a fundamental corporeal gap or strangeness, a unique situation which allows them to examine, experiment with and operate upon bodies (of themselves and others) in the first place (1971–1972, p. 20).

A congruent account was published by Francisco Varela (2001), who underwent a liver transplant and whose auto-ethnographical memoirs, published posthumously as *Intimate distances*, build on (and explicitly refer to) Nancy's essay. Again, the experience of intrusion is the core motif. After the operation, tubes, sutures and drains continue to cover the recipient's prostrate body from nose to pubic zone. He feels broken up, in bits and pieces. It is as if he is pregnant, carrying an infant inside his abdomen, revealed and monitored with the help of scanners and other optic devices. The sight of the new liver inside his body invokes in him "a mixture of intimacy and foreignness" (p. 260). He sees himself as a pioneer because, increasingly, individuals will be faced with circulating body parts, passing from one body to the next, redesigning the landscape of corporeal boundaries (p. 260). The "foreign" liver (p. 261) inside his body first of all confirms that the old liver had become foreign and alien to him, corroded by cirrhosis, something definitely "un-me" (p. 262). The new organ from now on beckons his attention. In the case of rejection, the cellular guardians known as lymphocytes (once the hallmark of Self-ness and intimacy) will have to be exterminated by toxic "napalm warfare". Transplantation has turned the body into an inevitable target of intrusions which are bound to become increasingly "obscene" (260). Still, notwithstanding its physical brutality, it is not the implantation technology *as such* which introduces alterity into the lived body. Rather, the technology slips into a foreignness which is already there, disclosing me-ness as a precarious condition from the very outset. The technology that opens him up, drowns him in anaesthetics, implants the ice-packed organ and eventually sutures him together again will never be something of the past. Rather, the gaping gap is bound to stay, inviting multiple new intrusions, from drug treatments (inducing diabetes, diarrhoea, anaemia and chronic fatigue) up to medical controls. Notwithstanding all efforts to rebuild the recipient again, his body remains a paragon of foreignness.

Lacan's notion extimacy seems to capture this post-operational way of being-in-the-world described by Nancy and Varela quite convincingly, notably because, in their accounts, extimacy surfaces not as a symptom connected to organ transfer specifically, but rather as an inherent dimension of human embodiment as such, which is highlighted rather than brought about by this experience. Rather than regarding the experience of the lived body in terms of wholeness as "primary", and the fragmented, composite body of science as "derivative" (Merleau-Ponty 1945), transplantation medicine discloses the extent to which fragmentation and alienation constitute a profound and primordial dimension of embodiment as such. And rather than being purely first-person accounts, these memoirs by Nancy and Varela stage dramatic dialogues between first person perspectives (voiced by recipients and focussed on the lived body) and third person perspectives (mediated by biomedical technology); between introspection and externalisation. And it is notably here that the added value of a Lacanian perspective (compared to the existing literature on embodiment) reveals itself. Whereas phenomenology starts from the primacy of the *lived* body, seeing techno-scientific biomedical representations of the body as derivative, other types of discourse (not only biomedicine itself, but also its supporting legal and bioethical superstructure) rather take the *objectified* body as its point of departure, that is: the body as dissected by anatomy, quantified by physiology, opened-up by ultrasonography and so on (Zwart 1998). Lacan, however, sees both dimensions of bodily existence as equally primordial, urging us to focus our attention on the inevitable ontological tensions and clashes between the two, on the evolving dialectic, emphasising that none of these versions of the body (neither the lived or first-person version, nor the techno-scientific or third-person version) can claim to capture the elusive *real* body, which only reveals itself in the folds and margins of these competing experiences of embodiment. Eventually, however, their dialectic proves an unequal interaction, as the first-person (or lived body) perspective finds itself time and again decentred by the powerful, intrusive, technological gaze. In the following chapters, this clash of basic experiences of the body will be analysed from an oblique perspective, exemplified by organ transplant cinema.

REFERENCES

Lacan, J. 1971–1972. *Le savoir du psychoanalyst* (unpublished seminar). http://www.valas.fr/.

Merleau-Ponty, M. 1945. *Phénoménologie de la perception*. Paris: Gallimard.

Nancy, J.-L. 2000/2010. *L'intrus*. Paris: Galilée.

Varela, F. 2001. Intimate Distances: Fragments for a Phenomenology of Organ Transplantation. *Journal of Consciousness Studies* 8 (5–7): 259–271.

Zwart, H. 1998. Medicine, Symbolization and the 'Real Body': Lacan's Understanding of Medical Science. *Medicine, Healthcare and Philosophy: A European Journal* 1 (2): 107–117.

CHAPTER 17

An Oblique Perspective: Organ Transplant Cinema

Abstract Movies involving organ procurement provide a window into the tensions and paradoxes of transplantation medicine. They constitute a different stage, an ontological laboratory, where the intriguing vicissitudes of the *lived* body, challenged by the intrusive *techno-scientific* body (and its ethical-legal support system) and frustrated by the recalcitrance of the elusive *real* body, may be analysed and assessed in profuse detail. Organ transplantation cinema zooms in on the violence and power relationships at work in procuring transplant organs. Transplantation movies consistently tend to problematise the ethical soundness of organ harvesting. The popularity of organ theft as a key cinematic motif (e.g. organ trafficking by criminal organisations) is symptomatic of this tendency.

Keywords Oblique perspective • Organ transplant cinema • Triangulation • Organ theft cinema • Genres of the imagination

As indicated earlier, movies involving organ procurement provide a window into the tensions and paradoxes of transplantation medicine. They constitute a different stage, an ontological laboratory, where the intriguing vicissitudes of the *lived* body, challenged by the intrusive *techno-scientific* body (and its ethical-legal support system: e.g. the bio-ethical grammar of informed consent etc.), and frustrated by the recalcitrance of the elusive *real* body, may be analysed and assessed in profuse detail. As

© The Author(s) 2019
H. A. E. Zwart, *Purloined Organs*,
https://doi.org/10.1007/978-3-030-05354-3_17

pointed out by Sharp (2006, 2007) and others, a basic tension can be discerned between the *base* of transplantation medicine (the corporeal—*corpo-real*—surgical realities) and its *superstructure* (the bioethical idiom of sharing, dignity and consent). The intrusive violence of transplantation as a corporeal practice is obfuscated by its persistent framing in terms of voluntary donation and restoration of integrity (Kass 1992; Awaya 1994; Scheper-Hughes 2000). Here, the oblique cinematic perspective may offer a different, revelatory viewpoint. In contrast to standardised university discourse, transplantation cinema focuses on the questionable origin of the organs at hand and on the violence and power relationships at work in procuring them. Transplantation cinema constitutes a genre in its own right and many examples of organ transplant movies can be given, but they rather consistently tend to problematise the ethical soundness of organ harvesting as such. The popularity of organ theft as a key cinematic motif (in movies depicting organ trafficking by criminal organisations) is a symptom of this tendency.

Contemporary movies about organ transplants provide valuable source material for analysing and assessing the ontological dimension of transplantation medicine, and this includes techno-thrillers and action movies about organised organ trafficking. They do not merely serve as "illustrations" of bioethical issues (Livingston 2006, p. 11; Schicktanz et al. 2010, p. 67), but rather provide a stage where emerging experiences of embodiment (and the discontents they give rise to) can be explored (Zwart 2015). Since Michael Crichton's movie *COMA* (released in 1978), in which healthy bodies are drugged and kept in comatose states until their organs can be removed for sale, a whole series of movies about organ commodification or even organ thefts have been released. They provide relevant input for analysing the ontological repercussions of the commodification of body parts (unleashed by transplantation medicine) and for addressing the question how transplantation medicine affects human subjectivity as such.

Methodologically speaking, the use of organ transplantation cinema constitutes an exercise in *triangulation*. Biomedical discourse (and this includes its bioethical and legal auxiliaries) is confronted with a different scene or stage—"Schauplatz", to use the Freudian term (1900/1942, p. 541)—where important aspects are brought to the fore which tend to be obfuscated and disavowed in normal university discourse. In university discourse, as we have seen, the biomedical (or bioethical) expert (S_2) takes the floor as *agent*, determined to tame and domesticate the allusive object *a*. What is obfuscated, first of all, is that this practice conveys a particular ontological understanding of the body (S_1) and, secondly, that the recalcitrant object (the liver in the case of Starzl) gives rise to experiences of suffering, frustration and despair ($ as by-product), not only on the part of organ recipients, but also among biomedical researchers (such as Starzl) themselves. Organ transplantation cinema allows us to take an anti-clockwise turn to the left, towards a different type of discourse, the *discourse of the analyst*, bracketing normal bioethical discourse (S_2) and focussing on the interaction between the *object* (*a*) and the *subject* ($) of desire, acknowledging that the object plays an active role, triggering the recipient's desire. For indeed, organ transplantation cinema frames organ transplants as objects of desire, as enigmatic things which incorporate promises of restitution. Procurable organs are things of value, apparently more valuable than life itself. To study how anxieties and uneasiness associated with organ transfer are enacted, three examples of organ transplant movies will be assessed, namely the Canadian movie *Jésus de Montréal* (1990), the French movie *L'Intrus* (2004) and the American movie *Crank 2: High Voltage* (2009). All three consistently address the intrusive dimension of transplantation medicine, highlighted by illicit organ procurement as a key symptom. An element of theft always seems involved, and this reflects the controversial nature of the ontological reframing of the human body as an aggregate of commodifiable and reusable items, brought about by transplantation medicine.

References

Awaya, T. 1994. The Theory of Neo-Cannibalism. *Japanese Journal of Philosophy* 3: 29–47.

Freud, S. 1900/1942. Die Traumdeutung. In *Gesammelte Werke II/III*. London: Imago.

Kass, L. 1992. Organs for Sale? Propriety, Property, and the Price of Progress. *The Public Interest* Spring (107): 65–86.

Livingston, P. 2006. Theses on Cinema as Philosophy. *The Journal of Aesthetics and Art Criticism* 64 (1): 11–18.

Scheper-Hughes, N. 2000. The Global Traffic in Human Organs. *Current Anthropology* 41: 191–224.

Schicktanz, S., C. Wiesemann, and S. Wöhlke. 2010. *Teaching Ethics in Organ Transplantation and Tissue Donation Cases and Movies*. Göttingen: Universitätsverlag.

Sharp, L. 2006. *Strange Harvest: Organ Transplants, Denatured Bodies and the Transformed Self.* Berkeley/Los Angeles/London: University of California Press.

———. 2007. *Bodies, Commodities and Biotechnologies. Death, Mourning and Scientific Desire in the Realm of Human Organ Transfer.* New York: Columbia University Press.

Zwart, H. 2015. A New Lease on Life: A Lacanian Analysis of Cognitive Enhancement Cinema. In *Handbook Posthumanism in Film and Television*, ed. Michael Hauskeller et al., 214–224. London: Palgrave Macmillan.

CHAPTER 18

Procuring the Gift

Abstract My first example (the French-Canadian movie *Jésus de Montréal* by Denis Arcand, released in 1990) is particularly telling because it enacts the bioethical concept of the gift. A group of young actors is invited to update and perform the story of the crucifixion of Christ at a Catholic sanctuary. From a Christian perspective, the integrity of the body can only be safeguarded if organ donation concurs with the concept of the Samaritan gift, as a gesture of charity and love, but this scheme is distorted by the relentless commodification of body parts. Once pronounced brain-dead, Daniel's procured organs allow the blind to see and the moribund to survive: theatre as a preparatory rehearsal for what biomedicine has in store for us. Yet, in a godless world, the hope of resurrection inevitably gives way to uneasiness about the manner in which the organs were procured.

Keywords Oblique perspective • Organ transplant cinema • Donorship • Consent • Christianity • Brain death • Beneficence

My first example, which I find particularly telling because initially it seems to enact the bioethical concept of the *gift*, is the French-Canadian movie *Jésus de Montréal*, written and directed by Denis Arcand and released in 1990. A group of young actors is invited to update and perform the story of the crucifixion of Christ at a Catholic sanctuary. Their convincing theatrical performance attracts many enthusiastic visitors, but upsets the

H. A. E. Zwart, *Purloined Organs*,
https://doi.org/10.1007/978-3-030-05354-3_18

religious authorities, represented by a local priest, who decides to interrupt the show just before it reaches its passionate climax: the dramatic death of Jesus on the cross. In the turmoil which unfolds, the heavy cross, with Daniel Coulombe (the actor playing Jesus) already attached to it, falls to the ground, and Daniel, badly wounded, is taken to an emergency ward. Initially, he seems to recover, but in an underground station he collapses once again. This time he is pronounced brain-dead, whereupon the doctors ask the two women accompanying him (playing the role of Mary and Mary of Magdalene) for his body—or rather, his organs. In the course of the movie, not only Jesus (Daniel Coulombe) himself, but also the other team members, although sceptical at first, increasingly identify themselves with their roles.

The connection between donorship, self-sacrifice and the story of Jesus builds on a long history (Zwart 2014) and becomes increasingly noticeable as the narrative unfolds. The actor's name is already an omen: the prophet Daniel as a prefiguration of Christ who, in the New Testament, is associated with a dove (*colombe* in French). Before being called to follow Him, the other actors had been forced to sell their bodies and voices in various ways (by starring in erotic commercials or dubbing pornography, for instance). Early on in the movie, a producer, spotting a young and handsome actor, exclaims "I want his head … for my advertisement campaign", a reference to John the Baptist, whose head serves as partial object in Christian iconography. The correspondences between movie and gospel quickly multiply. The theatrical performance makes Jesus come to life again as someone who allows the blind to see, revivifies the dead and eventually dies to repair human shortcomings. After the last (pizza) supper and the crucifixion scene, his disciples have lost the one thing which gave meaning to their lives, but by serving as an organ resource, Daniel becomes *flesh* again.

The movie also enacts a dramatic shift in terms of types of discourse. Initially, the focus is on the clash between divided, impetuous subjects (Daniel and the other actors: $) and the establishment (represented by the priest: S_1), in accordance with the structure of the hysteric's discourse. Instead of keeping their distance, these subjects (young actors who had been selling their bodies and voices, as targets of exploitation) throw themselves into their roles, but they do not really know what is driving their desire and their protests. Initially, the target of their protestation is the priest, for whom their performance seems too passionate, too disruptive. In a dialogue with Daniel (reminiscent of Dostoevsky's parable of the

Grand Inquisitor), the priest (who initially had offered him the assignment) explains his change of course by saying that Christianity provides consolation to the ill, the outcasts and the handicapped, but especially to those who cannot "afford Lacanian psychoanalysis". Daniel's performance threatens to disrupt this modest practice of beneficence.

The focus on the priest as their initial target of their protestation proves misguided, however. The contemporary world is no longer under the sway of a powerful church on the hunt for souls (as spiritual object *a*), but rather under the sway of biopower, more precisely: a technocratic system prowling for organs (the object *a* of transplantation medicine). After the dramatic turn (Daniel's second death on the cross), these objects of desire (*a*) come into view. The partial organs of Daniel and his disciples (their heads, their body parts, their procurable organs) is what commercialised cannibalism is really after. From a Christian perspective, the integrity of the body can only be safeguarded if organ donation concurs with the concept of the Samaritan gift as we have seen, as a gesture of charity and love (Zwart 2000), but this scheme is drastically distorted by the relentless commodification of body parts. Once pronounced brain-dead, Daniel's procured organs allow the blind to see and the moribund to survive: theatre as a preparatory rehearsal for what biomedicine has in store for us. Yet, in a godless world, the hope of resurrection inevitably gives way to uneasiness about the manner in which the organs were procured. Much more care and attention are given posthumously to Daniel's life-saving organs than to his injured body, and the informed consent procedure is questionable, to put it mildly. Daniel is exploited in various ways, but especially posthumously, when he is robbed of his organs. The evil voice which (in the beginning of the movie) signalled a desire for an actor's head now preys upon Daniel's body as a multiple-organ resource. But this, interestingly, has become a core motif in transplantation cinema as such.

References

Zwart, H. 2000. From Circle to Square: Integrity, Vulnerability and Digitalization. In *Bioethics and Law II: Four Ethical Principles*, ed. P. Kemp et al., 141–153. Copenhagen: Rhodos.

———. 2014. The Donor Organ as an 'Object A': A Lacanian Perspective on Organ Donation and Transplantation Medicine. *Medicine, Health Care & Philosophy: A European Journal* 17 (4): 559–571. https://doi.org/10.1007/s11019-014-9553-1.

CHAPTER 19

The Toxicity of the Purloined Implant

Abstract My second example of organ transplant cinema is the French movie *The Intruder*, directed by Clair Denis and released in 2004. The black market organ is not a life-saving item, but a toxic intrusion. Organ harvesting disrupts bodily integrity, for the donor as well as for the recipient, and this intrusive violence, concealed by standard transplantation discourse, surfaces in organ transplant cinema, with its symptomatic predilection for stories about illegal organ markets and organ theft. In movies, in other words, the ontological trauma is brought to the surface as a moral flaw.

Keywords Intrusion • Extimacy • Organ theft cinema • Organ traffic • Commodification

My second example of organ transplant cinema is the French movie *L'Intrus* (The Intruder), directed by Clair Denis, released in 2004 and inspired by Jean-Luc Nancy's eponymous essay discussed above. Although at first glance any noticeable connection between essay and movie seems missing, author and director are "in touch" with one another (Streiter 2008). *L'Intrus* tells the story of a retired businessman (who also seems to have been a secret agent) named Louis Trébor, living in a forest cabin near the French-Swiss Jura border and suffering from a heart condition. After a cardiac attack, he travels to Geneva (not coincidentally the capital of

H. A. E. Zwart, *Purloined Organs*,
https://doi.org/10.1007/978-3-030-05354-3_19

watchmaking) to buy himself a heart, procured on the black market with the help of a mysterious Russian woman, who continues to stalk him afterwards. He is plagued by uncanny dreams, moreover, one of which involves a heart which, apparently, has just been torn from a body, and is now dropped in a snow-clad landscape, where it is eaten by dogs (who perform the role of lymphocytes: detecting and preventing intrusions).

With a cocktail of medicines in his luggage, Louis abandons lovers, dogs, son and grandchildren to embark on an odyssey which takes him via Pusan (South Korea) and Papeete (Tahiti) to the Marquis islands, which he visited long ago as a young man, in search of an abandoned son he never met, and who eventually seems non-existent. Implant surgery fails to fend off death, however. In these desolate/paradisiac surroundings, his body persists in rejecting the implanted organ and his health quickly deteriorates, while local inhabitants organise an impromptu casting session to provide him with a substitute "son", on whom he desires to bestow his fortune, provided the latter agrees to accompany him during his final voyage home.

Instead of mimicking Jean-Luc Nancy's essay, the movie seems to reverse it. For instance, instead of patiently waiting for the arrival of an available organ (provided via legal channels), Louis Trébor (an inconsiderate, selfish man of action) immediately takes his fate into his own hands by choosing the "treatment of urgency". Via the Internet, he contacts an obscure Russian organisation specialised in organ trafficking. Instead of pondering over the contingencies of life (as Varela did), Louis buys an expensive illegal heart, with suspicious cash money stashed in a Swiss safe. As Nancy (2005) phrases it, who actually wrote an analysis of the movie, in order to keep death from intruding into his life (via the faltering organ), Louis calls upon life (the implanted organ) to interrupt the process of ageing and dying.

As soon as the implant is grafted, however, Louis noticeably begins to age. The implant is not a "restitution of integrity" (Nancy 2000/2010, 2005), but a toxic substance, a "gift" indeed, insofar as *gift* means both "donation" (English) and "poison" (German) in Germanic languages. Instead of rejuvenation, his body suffers from intrusion and rejection. The Russian woman who stalks her toxic "gift" seems the personification of his guilty conscience seeking atonement: the "exteriorisation" of his illicit implant (Sweeney 2005). He tries to outrun his fate, to camouflage himself, but to no avail. When he implores her to stop dogging him, in view of his heart problems, she replies that his heart is not ill, but *empty*. As the neo-organ is rejected, a fatal emptiness or vacuole re-emerges, but Louis is also "heartless" in a figurative sense. The Russian woman (his voice of conscience), demands penitence (a "change of heart"), like in a medieval morality play.

The illegal transaction, meant to offer "a new lease on life" (Zwart 2015), proves a Faustian Pact (Beugnet 2008). The black market organ (the object *a*) is not a life-saving item, but a toxic intrusion, notwithstanding medication, Korean massage (by a blind masseuse), long-distance travel and other instances of denial. The movie stresses the questionable or even unsettling origin of implants and the problematic nature of organ procurement from an ontological (depth ethical) point of view. Organ harvests involve intrusions of bodily integrity, for the donor as well as for the recipient, and this intrusive violence, concealed by normal transplantation discourse (as a sub-branch of university discourse), surfaces in organ transplant cinema, with its symptomatic predilection for stories about illegal organ markets and organ theft. In movies, in other words, the obfuscated ontological trauma is brought to the surface as a moral flaw.

This is emphasised quite explicitly towards the end of *L'Intrus* where it is suggested that Louis' new heart was actually procured from the body of his abandoned, natural, French son, whose corpse (with a chest roughly sewn up) is found deposited in a morgue—by the Russian organ mafia perhaps, who apparently played a draconic joke on Louis. The French son's corpse is taken on board as well, joining the moribund father on his final voyage—or is Louis rather on his way to his next heart implant?

In Lacanian terms, the faltering heart is the extimate object of concern (*a*). Organs (initially concealed within living corporeal flesh) are singled out by the biomedical gaze, first of all to determine their place and function (think, for instance, of classroom anatomical models from which organs, painted in distinguishable colours, can be taken out, until the body is completely emptied). As Merleau-Ponty (1945) pointed out, the lived body collapses as soon as it is cast as an object of science. As soon as the biomedical gaze detects Louis' cardiac condition, his body becomes marked by a stigma of loss, and this intensifies his position as a craving subject ($\$$), in frantic search of a life-saving, extimate, detachable, implantable object ($\$ \lozenge a$). The latter becomes an obsession to which everything else is sacrificed (even his son). The new heart becomes an object of desire, meant to redress a basic deficiency. Building on Aristophanes' myth in *Symposium*, Lacan refers to this experience of loss as a "lamella": an ultra-thin, sharp surface (1964/1973, p. 222) which separates us from a part of ourselves (in this case, the faltering heart), bringing about a cut, a wound, a scar, creating an orifice, an erogenous zone, separating the subject from something to which he seems entitled and which he cannot do without. The loss $(-\varphi)$ becomes a vector, relentlessly pointing towards the missing (allegedly life-saving, but actually quite toxic and intrusive) object a. It cannot be just any heart, moreover, for this time it should match, and towards the end of the movie, as we have seen, it is suggested that the implant was procured from Louis' own son, whose heart now lives on inside his chest, while he himself is sailing towards his "second death". Perhaps his son's heart became his unique object of desire because of a belief that this organ would not fail him, would prove compatible, would not be rejected.

Again, an element of Christology is at work here, as is emphasised by Nancy (2005) and others (Streiter 2008; Morrey 2008a, b). The gruesome scar on Louis' chest (a brusque reminder of the intrusive organ: Sweeney 2005) is a partial cross and in the Gospels Jesus Himself is cast as the sacrificed son, who is resurrected via the father. Together (father, sacrificed son and transplant organ) represent a trinity, but the Death of God obscures the horizon, so that Louis must face damnation: he is sent on his final voyage towards his "second" death (Apocalypse, 2:11; 20:6; 20:14). In *L'Intrus*-the-movie, we have entered the right panel of Bosch's triptych, where gruesome instruments are employed to maltreat, dissect, dismember and dismantle bodies (both of donors and of recipients). What is initially obfuscated, but systematically disclosed (in a dispassionate, clinical, step-by-step manner) in *L'Intrus* is the awareness that the discourse of bodily integrity and benevolent donation on which transplantation discourse (as an instance of university discourse) builds, functions as a screen and eclipses a disconcerting truth, namely the transformation of body parts into commodities, into things for sale, or even theft (Fig. 19.1).

I will now turn to my third case study, *Crank 2: High Voltage*, a "lowbrow" action movie about organised organ theft released in 2009: a

Normal biomedical / bioethical discourse (S$_2$): organ transplantation as restitution of normalcy	The domestication of the procurable and implantable organ (a)
The disavowed truth (S$_1$): replacing the ontology of the gift by the ontology of commodification and recycling	By-products: from the intrusive scar to victims of organ trafficking ($\$$)

Fig. 19.1 Organ transplantation: University discourse

contemporary cinematic enactment of the sardonic right panel of Bosch's triptych. What emerges as a sinister and disconcerting truth in the previous two examples is now blatantly embraced, as a symptom of the zeitgeist: the human body has now irretrievably lost its coherence.

REFERENCES

Beugnet, M. 2008. The Practice of Strangeness: L'Intrus – Claire Denis (2004) and Jean-Luc Nancy (2000). *Film-Philosophy* 12 (1): 31–48.

Lacan, J. 1964/1973. *Le séminaire de Jacques Lacan XI: Les quatre concepts fondamentaux de la psychanalyse.* Paris: Éditions du Seuil.

Merleau-Ponty, M. 1945. *Phénoménologie de la perception.* Paris: Gallimard.

Morrey, D. 2008a. Introduction: Claire Denis and Jean-Luc Nancy. *Film-Philosophy* 12 (1): i–vi.

———. 2008b. Open Wounds: Body and Image in Jean-Luc Nancy and Claire Denis. *Film-Philosophy* 12 (1): 10–31.

Nancy, J.-L. 2000/2010. *L'intrus.* Paris: Galilée.

———. 2005. *L'Intrus selon Claire Denis.* Remue.net: http://remue.net/spip.php?article679.

Streiter, A. 2008. The Community According to Jean-Luc Nancy and Claire Denis. *Film-Philosophy* 12 (1): 49–62.

Sweeney, R.E. 2005. The Hither Side of Solutions: Bodies and Landscape in *L'Intrus. Senses of Cinema* 36. http://sensesofcinema.com/2005/feature-articles/intrus/.

Zwart, H. 2015. A New Lease on Life: A Lacanian Analysis of Cognitive Enhancement Cinema. In *Handbook Posthumanism in Film and Television,* ed. Michael Hauskeller et al., 214–224. London: Palgrave Macmillan.

CHAPTER 20

Crank 2: High Voltage, or the Purloined Organ

Abstract My third case study is *Crank 2: High Voltage*, a low-brow action movie about organised organ theft released in 2009, revolving around an organ hunt. What is acted-out in the movie is the experience that transplantation medicine turns the hero's organs into objects of desire. Partial organs become objects of desire for craving subjects: notably men on the wane. Bodies are organic containers for valuable, detachable, commodifiable objects, transportable in Styrofoam coolers. The purloined organ turns up unexpectedly, is more often absent than present and may show up in very unlikely places. It is unique and priceless, but at the same time replaceable by electronic substitutes, and a most dangerous thing to have.

Keywords Organ theft cinema • Extimacy • Implants • Objects of desire • Organ traffic

At the start of the movie, male protagonist Chev Chelios (a.k.a "Superman") is thrown out of a helicopter and hit by a car. After landing on asphalt somewhere in Los Angeles, the camera zooms in on his empty gaze: he seems definitely brain dead and his body is promptly picked up and transported to a clandestine DIY operation unit inside a brothel, where his organs will be harvested, his heart to begin with: that which makes him "tick". Instruments for measuring blood level (mmHg), heart rate (ECG) and oxygen saturation (SaO_2) come into view. The removal of

© The Author(s) 2019
H. A. E. Zwart, *Purloined Organs*,
https://doi.org/10.1007/978-3-030-05354-3_20

Chelios' (hyper-normal) heart mimics a delivery scene. A Caesarean-like section is performed with a razor-sharp lamella and the procured organ is lifted high into the air to be gazed at in admiration: something highly valuable, about to start a new life. The surgeons seem like Aztec priests, with prostitutes flanking them as operation assistants/priestesses, gazing in awe at the famous organ (φ), naked and unveiled.[1]

At a certain point during the operation, Chelios awakens for a brief moment to see what is going on. An artificial (electronic) heart is implanted as replacement. The second organ on the list, already marked for removal, is his penis. Both organs are considered key condensations of his identity. He manages to escape just in time, however, with a yellow box attached to his body: an external battery pack to keep his artificial heart going. In psychoanalysis, this is known as displacement: a shift of focus from phallus to heart, while the latter is sacrificed to rescue the former. Realising that his chest has been emptied (that a vacuole has been created), the remainder of the movie is a chaotic, high-pace journey through murky, multi-ethnic metropolitan quarters, inhabited by sex workers and criminal gangs, in pursuit of his heart (to be re-implanted as soon as possible). In Lacanian grammar, the movie reflects the matheme of desire ($\$ \lozenge a$), with Chelios, the damaged Superman ($\cancel{A}$) desperately trying to restore his lost integrity ($\cancel{A} + a = 1$) by retrieving and re-embedding an impossible lost object. Via his cell phone, Chelios contacts a friend, a former heart surgeon who offers him a crash course in cardiac surgery and implantation medicine.

As a result of yet another car crash, however, the external battery is damaged, so that a new dimension is added to the search for his heart: Chelios is in need of electricity to prevent his ersatz organ from faltering (electricity = life). Rather than a seat of emotions, the heart is a source (as well as a voracious consumer) of electric energy. Various items serve as ersatz electricity providers: car batteries, skin-to-skin friction (by his ex-girlfriend) and (eventually) an overhead high-voltage cable (Chelios desperately climbs a pole that carries the cable and is electrocuted: the movie's crucifixion scene). The purloined heart, deposited in a white Styrofoam cooler, is carried off by a crook, but when Chelios manages to retrieve the box it proves empty: the purloined organ has disappeared once again (a). It has already been implanted inside the chest of an elderly gangster who,

---

[1] Notice that the shift of focus from *foetus* and *phallus* to "something else" (the heart) as object *a* (and from *delivery* and *castration* to *organ procurement*) exemplifies what in psychoanalysis is known as *metonymy* or *displacement*.

with the help of this powerful supplement (although still on the waiting list for Chelios' penis) experiences a new lease on life, a surge of *jouissance*, as a prostitute client. He is seduced, however, by the former surgeon's girlfriend (herself a former sex worker) and lured into a makeshift operation room, where the purloined heart is finally restored to its rightful owner—although it remains unclear whether Chelios will survive his taxing adventures.

Crank 2: High Voltage is a cinematic remake of the *Frankenstein* motif. Electricity = life and the human body is an aggregate of replaceable parts (the Frankenstein *philosopheme*). Transplantation surgery has become common-place by now and is proliferating into garage surgery. On various occasions, notably at the beginning and end of the movie, Chelios (resting on an operating table) unexpectedly opens his eyes, as if a body that was supposed to be (brain-) dead is suddenly brought back to life again, as in the *Frankenstein* story. Unlike Frankenstein's Monster, however, who acts as the recipient of *other* people's organs, Chelios is himself the resource from which highly valuable parts are procured. And while Frankenstein's Monster prefers a snow-clad landscape, Chelios' body is continuously heated up. His name contains a reference to the solar deity *Helios*, the ultimate source of energy, to which the letter C is added, the first letter of the title *Crank*, the signifier which 'carries' the movie. The word *Cranky* means "bizarre" and *crank* may refer to an eccentric person, obsessed with bizarre objectives (such as retrieving a purloined organ). A "crank", in other words, is a *craving subject ($)* par excellence. In German, *krank* means ill (as in *Krankengeschichte*), while to *crank up* means to enhance someone (as in the case of hyper-normal, "cranked-up" athletes).

The detachable heart is the movie's object *a*, put into circulation from one body to the next, as a source of jouissance, but also as a life-threatening intruder, for whoever happens to be carrying it. Chelios' heart and penis are not the only detachable body parts, however. Other examples of corporeal items that come off are the tip of an elbow (sliced off from a male body with the help of a knife), nipples removed from the breast of a (heavily tattooed) gangster and the silicone breasts of a transvestite sex worker (hit by bullets during a gun fight in a striptease bar). Bodies do not count for much: they are treated as throw-away items, easily replaceable, in line with the right panel of Bosch's triptych, which likewise depicts an underground world of brothel sex, excessively violent combats and sadistic corporeal punishments, where human bodies are tortured, penetrated and dismembered. The corpses of gangsters and sex workers pile up as the story unfolds, and much more value is placed on removable body *parts* than on bodies as such. This notably applies to partial organs that may function as ersatz objects such as hearts, breasts, nipples and phalluses. When the tip of an elbow (severed from the body with the help of a machete) falls to the floor, it actually looks like a miniature version of a cut off breast.

The yellow battery pack attached to Chelios' chest likewise acts as a (life-saving but unreliable) substitute object *a*: an electronic, ready-at-hand replacement. This also goes for the hero's cell phone, an electronic umbilical cord connecting him with the voice of the life-saving Other (the former surgeon) who provides him with vital instruction on how to survive organ theft and energy loss.

The manhunt is actually an organ hunt. What is acted-out in the movie is the experience that partial organs have become objects of desire for craving subjects: men on the wane, such as elderly gangsters (*$ ◊ a*). Bodies are organic containers for valuable, detachable, commodifiable objects, transportable in Styrofoam coolers. Transplantation medicine has turned the hero's heart into an object of desire, conveying the promise that singular forms of *jouissance* (earthly delights) will be within reach once it is implanted (STEAL ME!). The purloined organ functions as the movie's object *a*, turning up unexpectedly, being more often absent (*Fort*) than present (*Da*). It is hardly ever where it is expected to be and may show up in very unlikely places. It is unique and priceless, but at the same time replaceable by electronic substitutes, and a most dangerous thing to have.

As for the ethnic dimension, a white male hero becomes the target of an organ hunt organised by Asian gangster, so that white, male organs are presented as the most valuable items on the global market. This concurs with how organ theft is enacted in other organ theft movies. *Turistas* for instance involves a group of affluent young American tourists backpacking through the Brazilian jungle. After being drugged on a paradisiac beach, they fall into the hands of an organ harvesting ring. In an improvised operation room somewhere in a tropical forest, a white female patient wakes up for a brief moment, vaguely aware of her predicaments. The gang actually claims moral-political motives. Rich tourists come to Brazil for organs and sex, they argue, exploiting human bodies, but now the tables are turned, so that the bodies of young tourists are used as organ resource. The main villain is a biomedical Robin Hood, stealing organs from the rich to hand them over to the poor (uninsured craving patients in a public hospital in Rio de Janeiro). This reversal is symptomatic, for in real life, organ traffic tends to be fairly one-directional, with organs consistently travelling from poorer regions of the world towards the organ-hungry affluent West, notably the U.S., the U.K. and Israel (Declaration of Istanbul 2008). That organ theft cinema reverses this scheme may be taken as an instance of denial, a mechanism of defence, a symptom of anxiety and guilt produced by global inequality. Still, in the end (after a series of implausible escapes), most of the allegedly helpless tourists manage to survive, with their Caucasian organs still in place.

Reference

Declaration of Istanbul on Organ Trafficking and Transplant Tourism. 2008. *Kidney International* 74 (7): 854–859.

CHAPTER 21

Depth Ethics and the Oblique Perspective

Abstract Transplantation medicine profoundly affects experiences of embodiment, notably through the commodification of body parts. There is an intrusive, dehumanising dimension to organ procurement which tends to be obfuscated by a moral discourse shrouded in denial. Yet, what is concealed (repressed) on the manifest level of discourse is bound to resurge in organ transplant cinema. The idea that commodification will solve the problem of organ scarcity by emptying the waiting lists is illusory. Although overcoming organ scarcity has become a mantra in the current debate, it eclipses the extent to which organ demand is actually constantly produced by transplantation medicine itself.

Keywords Denial • Organ transplant cinema • Organ procurement • Donation • Codicils

Transplantation medicine profoundly affects experiences of embodiment, notably through the commodification of body parts. There is an intrusive, dehumanising dimension to organ procurement which tends to be obfuscated by a moral discourse shrouded in euphemistic "denial" (Sharp 2006, p. 13). Yet, what is concealed (repressed) on the manifest level of discourse is bound to resurge in organ transplant cinema. This explains why organ transplantation provides "rich fodder for plots in a wide range of media, including thriller fiction, television dramas, and film" (Sharp 2006, p. 1).

In a famous scene from Monty Python's *The Meaning of Life*, procurement officials arrive at the home of a person who had signed a donor card, demanding his liver ("a large, eh, glandular, reddish-brown organ in your abdomen"). When he refuses to cooperate, they force their way into his house and drag him into the kitchen, where the precious item is taken out. This parody conveys a kernel of truth, giving voice to subliminal unease. Transplantation movies persistently focus on the problematic, dubious origin of donor organs. An element of theft and intrusion always seems involved: a symptom of the ontological uneasiness entailed in the reframing of the human body as an aggregate of replaceable and reusable items. The ensuing violence affects the donor's body first of all, but spills over to the recipient as well, hooked up to arrays of machines and subjected to poisonous pharmaceutical regimes. In Lacanian terms, the *real* intrusive violence of organ transfer is concealed both by *imaginary* portrayals of restored integrity and by the *symbolic* grammar of ownership, donation and informed consent. The paradoxical message of organ theft cinema, however, is that, to the extent that transplantation medicine becomes increasingly successful, human beings begin to fear for their organs. Medical progress comes with a price: the wholeness of the body is disrupted as organs become detachable items, displaying "commodity candidacy" (Appadurai 1986) as a basic feature.

In other words, commodification turns organs into potential market commodities, so that the buying and selling of organs becomes a prominent issue on the global bioethical agenda. Critics argue that the idea of organs for sale not only undermines the dignity of the human body, but also encourages the exploitation of the global poor, who are actually forced to sell their organs to affluent recipients in Western countries. Others, however, see an "eBay for organs" as a viable alternative to increase the number of available options, allowing transplant surgeons to save the lives of moribund recipients on waiting lists.

From a Lacanian perspective, the debate on transplantation medicine is played out on three levels. On the *symbolic* level, we are confronted with quantitative data about waiting lists and survival rates, but also with ethical justifications and moral procedures for obtaining informed consent, resulting in a Yes or No. Symbolisation is bent on *digitalisation*, on implementing clear, acknowledged dichotomies between "admissible" and "inadmissible" (Zwart 1998; Zwart and Hoffer 1998). On the *imaginary* level, we are faced with a Gestalt-switch, as ailing, moribund patients suddenly become happy and healthy, due to their organ implants, persuading audiences to enlist as donors. There is a third dimension, however, the dimension of the *real*, obfuscated as a rule, where both the moral accept-ability and the medical benefits of organ transfer become decidedly less clear-cut. Procurable organs are objects of desire, promising a new lease on life, but as object *a*, donor organs will thwart our expectations. Some health problems may be (partially) addressed, but new challenges and new intrusions are likely to arrive. In view of the high-paced developments in transplantation medicine, the demand for human organs tends to become insatiable. The idea that commodification will "solve" the problem of organ scarcity by "emptying" the waiting lists (Erin and Harris 2003; Hurst 2015) is illusory. Although overcoming "organ scarcity" has become a "mantra" in the current debate (Scheper-Hughes 2000), it eclipses the extent to which organ demand is actually constantly produced by trans-plantation medicine itself ($ as by-product). To the extent that more organs will become available, the number of potential recipients is bound to increase as well, in accordance with the matheme of desire ($ \lozenge a$).

References

Appadurai, A. 1986. *The Social Life of Things*. New York: Cambridge University Press.

Erin, C., and J. Harris. 2003. An Ethical Market in Human Organs. *Journal of Medical Ethics* 29: 137–138.

Hurst, S. 2015. The Ethics of Selling Body Parts. In *New Cannibal Markets: Globalization and Commodification of the Human Body*, ed. J.-D. Rainhorn and S. Boudamoussi, 47–56. Paris: Maison des sciences de l'homme.

Scheper-Hughes, N. 2000. The Global Traffic in Human Organs. *Current Anthropology* 41: 191–224.

Sharp, L. 2006. *Strange Harvest: Organ Transplants, Denatured Bodies and the Transformed Self*. Berkeley/Los Angeles/London: University of California Press.

Zwart, H. 1998. Medicine, Symbolization and the 'Real Body': Lacan's Understanding of Medical Science. *Medicine, Healthcare and Philosophy: A European Journal* 1 (2): 107–117.

Zwart, H., and C. Hoffer. 1998. *Orgaandonatie en lichamelijke integriteit*. Best: Damon.

CHAPTER 22

Encore: *Middlesex* and the Re-makeable Body

Abstract This final chapter shifts the focus to extimate (partial, intimate, external) organs (such as penises and breasts) which, standing out from the rest of the body, indicate gender identity, but may (for various reasons) seem unconvincing, detachable or misplaced. Surgical practices have evolved which aim to alter erogenous bodily parts, adapting them to societal expectations or individual desires, fuelled by the conviction that such partial objects can be refashioned, restored or remade. This will be addressed from an oblique perspective, focussing on three key sources, namely a famous tale reported by Plato, a Victorian case history analysed by Michel Foucault and a novel entitled *Middlesex* by Jeffrey Eugenides.

Keywords Modifiable bodies • Aristophanes • Hermaphroditism • Intersex • Gender • Nature and nurture • Acting-out • Working-through

So far, we have extensively explored how the experience of bodily fragmentation (the idea that partial objects can be added, refashioned or removed) was reinforced by transplantation medicine. This final chapter shifts the focus to extimate (partial, intimate, external) organs (such as penises and breasts) which, standing out from the rest of the body, indicate gender identity, but may (for various reasons) seem unconvincing, detachable or misplaced. Surgical practices have evolved which aim to alter

© The Author(s) 2019
H. A. E. Zwart, *Purloined Organs,*
https://doi.org/10.1007/978-3-030-05354-3_22

erogenous bodily parts, adapting them to societal expectations or individual desires, fuelled by the conviction that such partial objects can be refashioned, restored or remade. Rather than focusing on issues such as the "transgender epidemic" (i.e. the dramatic growth of individuals, especially teens, who are questioning their gender identity), or breast or penis enlargement surgery, I will zoom in on a phenomenon which was traditionally known as hermaphroditism, but which is currently discussed under biomedical headings such as *Disorders of Sex Development* (DSD), although outside the biomedical literature other labels (notably "intersex") are propagated. Basically, the discussion revolves around the question whether, why and when perceived gender-related "organ deficiencies" or misplacements should be surgically corrected. After introducing the issue, I will flesh out an oblique perspective, focussing on three key sources, namely: (a) a famous tale reported by Plato and already briefly referred to earlier; (b) a Victorian case history analysed by Michel Foucault; and (c) an intersex novel entitled *Middlesex* by Greek-American author Jeffrey Eugenides (2002/2003).

In history, mythology and art, hermaphrodites are individuals endowed with both male and female reproductive organs. In the current biomedical literature, the acronym DSD has been introduced to refer to genital, gonadal and/or chromosomal "ambiguity" or, more precisely, to "congenital conditions in which the development of chromosomal, gonadal or anatomical sex is atypical" (Lee et al. 2006). DSD covers a wide range of conditions and may be due to a broad variety of factors ranging from Tetrasomy X syndrome, XXYY syndrome, Turner syndrome and Klinefelter syndrome up to virilisation of 46 XX individuals or under-virilisation of 46 XY individuals. Although most of these conditions are considered rare, exact frequencies are a matter of dispute since prevalence depends on how exactly DSD is defined (Domurat Dreger 1998).

The label DSD is controversial. At the 2006 *Consensus Conference on Management of Intersex Disorders,* it was recommended that, from now on, DSD should be adopted to replace "potentially confusing and stigmatizing terms such as intersex, pseudo-hermaphroditism, hermaphroditism and sex reversal, as well as gender-based diagnostic labels such as male/female pseudo-hermaphroditism". Increasingly, however, DSD (as an allegedly more neutral heading) has been criticised as well, notably because it sees these phenomena as disorders. Wiesemann et al. (2010) therefore recommend the use of "less pathologizing" terms such as "*differences* in sex development" or "intersex"—a viewpoint shared by many patient organisations. Yet, allegedly neutral or less offensive labels often prove no less controversial than the ones they are meant to replace, a phenomenon known in psychoanalysis as metonymy or displacement. The uneasiness in coining an adequate label is symptomatic for the dilemmas and concerns involved.

Psychoanalytically speaking, intersex involves the presence, absence or (perceived) deficiency of erogenous partial organs associated with gender identity and reproduction. At birth, sex assignment of new-borns is based on genital morphological appearance, but also on chromosomal information (XX vs. XY). Until recently, it was common practice to assign sex identity shortly after birth and implement therapies (early corrective surgery) to restore (near) normal appearance, in combination with hormone therapy, adapting ambiguous genitals as closely as possible to assigned identity. This practice has become increasingly controversial, however, as patients and patient organisations indicate dissatisfaction with long-term outcomes of such decisions and challenge dichotomous interpretations of sex identity in terms of either/or. Physicians and health care providers themselves have also begun to question this practice and to consider alternatives. Critics see early corrective surgery as mutilation and recommend a moratorium on organ removal/adaptation until the individuals themselves can decide what they want their genitals to look like (Kipnis and Diamond 1998; Beh and Diamond 2000).

Intersex phenomena challenge the male-female divide as a basic component of the symbolic order. The male-female divide is firmly embedded in grammar, legal practices and cultural conventions. Sex identity is often the first distinctive feature we notice in others. It is the first question commonly asked when a baby is born and it significantly influences how we communicate and interact with one another. Already at a very early age, young children categorise family members, neighbours, visitors and passers-by (children as well as adults) in terms of male or female. Documents such as passports, birth announcements and dress codes confirm this fundamental distinction, cutting humanity into two more-or-less equal halves. Lacan (1966, p. 499) explains the functioning of the symbolic order by referring to public lavatories (ladies/gents) in restaurants, airports and train stations. We are expected to recognise immediately which of the two icons applies to us, resulting in a relentless "segregation" of the public sphere (1966, p. 500). Lacan adds an anecdote about two children discussing whether the train station they arrive at is called LADIES or GENTS. Gender segregation is part of our language, reflecting how in the distant past, sexual identity was bestowed not only on humans, but on many other things as well (mountains, trees, celestial bodies, etc. were seen as either male or female) and the current trend towards de-sexualisation, notably in academic and political circles (advocated by feminist authors and others since the 1970s and 1980s) is something many language users still struggle with.

And yet, the awareness that things are less straightforward than neat symbolic dichotomies suggest has been voiced since time immemorial. Hermaphroditism has been described from ancient times up to the present, challenging the idea that humankind can be easily split into two sections: girls and boys, women and men. All kinds of tensions and complications may arise when we try to connect the *symbolic* (the male-female divide as inscribed in legal, linguistic and cultural conventions) with the *real* (physical, experiential and behavioural) dimensions of embodiment.

Perhaps the most intriguing philosophical discussion of hermaphroditism was preserved in Plato's dialogue *Symposium*, written in the fourth century B.C. (around 380): a philosophical classic and literary masterpiece also known as *The Banquet*. When Aristophanes (the genius of Athenian comedy) is given the floor, he captures the origin of human sexual identity in a myth. Our original nature was by no means the same as it is now, he assures his audience. Initially, there were three types of human beings: males, females and hermaphrodites, although the latter is nowadays preserved mainly as a name of reproach. Their form was globular: each had four arms, four legs and two faces on a cylindrical neck, until Zeus proposed to slice them in two, just as eggs are sliced in two with a hair. Apollo subsequently turned their faces around and pulled their skin together, while Zeus moved their privy parts to the front, so that there might be conception and continuation of their kind (189E–191C). On closer inspection, this (at first sight rather bizarre) narrative proves highly interesting for various reasons. It evidently challenges the division of humankind into two stable categories, suggesting that sexual identity is the outcome of a complicated intervention which happened in a distant past. It also suggests the possibility of a third, intermediate, androgynous form. In short, human sexual identity is far from self-evident, but the outcome of a *surgical* operation, performed by Zeus. Sexual identity is enforced upon us, brought about by surgical means, by slicing human beings in two, like eggs, while our genitals were moved to the front. Bodily integrity is violated from the very beginning, and our bodies carry the scars of this traumatic experience. Sexual identity is something we have to adapt to, psychologically as well as physically, while modern individuals who display symptoms of sexual ambiguity seem straight descendants of these bisexual ancestors.

Zeus, the supreme deity, is the founder of the symbolic order who decides that there should be only two sexes, male and female, identifiable on the basis of their genitals. Subsequently, Apollo (the god of medicine) tries to make this work out in practice. Human bodies had to recover from an intrusive physical event, directed at the presence, absence and position of their genitals.

The operation performed by two deities reflects what is happening to us humans during prenatal intrauterine development and at birth. If we translate the language of myth into a biomedical vocabulary, what is described here is a process of meiosis (splitting), recombination and embryonic intrauterine unfolding and repositioning of various bodily parts: complicated processes that are part of our natural pre-natal development. The splitting already occurs at a moment when the embryo is in an egg-shaped phase. Subsequently, a series of dramatic developments unfolds. The morale of the story is that sexual identity is not something that can be taken for granted, but the outcome of a series of hazardous transformations taking place in a distant past (i.e. during embryonic and foetal episodes of existence) while the result may well remain problematic and ambiguous later in life. Notably at birth, surgeons and care takers (following in the footsteps of Apollo) may be faced with challenging questions, such as whether a surgical intervention, directed at restoring sexual identity and reconstructing bodily parts is warranted. In the case of genital ambiguity, the scars of the hazardous operation (unfolding during embryonic development) are more prominently visible than in normal cases, but they are never completely absent. The story also entails a *moral* message, namely that bodily integrity is not a primordial state of intactness, but something which is challenged from the very outset; endangered or even damaged almost by definition. Notably, there is something about human genitals, more than any other bodily part, that invokes a sense of vulnerability or out-of-place-ness.

Echoes of Aristophanes' story can be found in psychoanalysis. In *Beyond the pleasure principle* (1920/1940), Freud explicitly refers to it, arguing that, since science (university discourse) has so little to offer when it comes to explaining the origins of human sexuality, this deficiency may be complemented by consulting genres of the imagination, such as myths (p. 62).

Freud points out, moreover, that Aristophanes' version builds on even more ancient sources, such as the Upanishads, where it is explained that Atman was originally as large as a man and a woman intimately embracing one another. Suffering from loneliness, however, his body split up into two parts, male and female, but since the male body was only a half, the empty part had to be supplemented by the body of a woman and vice versa. Thus, men and women are like partial objects to each other, bodily halves separated from a primordial androgynous gigantic proto-body before birth.

Another variant can be found in *Genesis*, where God initially created a male, but decided to fashion a woman as well, from Adam's "rib", although the Hebrew word for rib may also mean "side" (Reik 1960). Notwithstanding the various versions of what seems a common archetypal script, the genesis of sexual identity is consistently presented as the outcome of a hazardous *surgical* intervention. We are told that Adam was put to sleep, as if God applied anaesthesia before the operation.

My second source is the case history of Alexina Barbin, presented by Michel Foucault (1978). According to Foucault, Alexina's case represents the Victorian approach of sexual identity in terms of normalcy and deviation which was also taken up by professional biomedicine. The Victorian preoccupation with normalcy was complemented, however, by a fascination with otherness. Alexina's memoirs were discovered after he/she committed suicide in Paris in 1868. Excerpts were published by the French physician Auguste Ambroise Tardieu[1] in his book *Question médico-légale de l'identité* (1872) and republished by Michel Foucault, more than a century later, in the context of his research into the history of sexuality.

At birth, Alexina was identified as female and she spent the larger part of her youth in boarding schools for girls. In a world almost exclusively inhabited by girls and women, she finally became a boarding school teacher herself. Here, a clandestine intimate relationship evolved between a female colleague and herself. As Alexina phrases it, it felt like a "sword of Damocles" suspended above her head (Foucault 1978, p. 75). She sensed an insurmountable distance between herself and others: as if she illegally

[1] Tardieu was a famous, albeit controversial, author in his own time. One of his earlier publications (1857) is generally regarded as the first scientific forensic report of child abuse. According to Masson (1984/2003), it served as an important source of information for Freud's 'seduction theory' (regarding sexual abuse during early childhood as causal factor in hysteria), which he later replaced by the conviction that most of these reports by patients during therapeutic sessions actually build on phantasies.

occupied a position not lawfully hers. Her discontent was aggravated by reading Ovid's *Metamorphoses*. She felt like a puny "Achilles" hiding in dormitories occupied by women (many of whom later took their vows to enter religious life) at a time when virginity was of utmost importance to the girls in question.

Because of severe abdominal complaints, she was sent to a physician, who examined her genitals but, in adherence to the principle of discretion, decided to remain silent. Alexina then made a full confession to a priest, who advised her to submit herself to a more extensive anatomical examination, which lead to a *Gestalt*-switch. All of a sudden, the organs which until then had been regarded as female were now suddenly redefined as male. A gross mistake had been made at birth and her sex should be reassigned. She was to take up a male position in society, to which she was now legally entitled. She suddenly became a man. Unable to find a suitable profession, however, she suffered from social exclusion and asphyxiated herself. Upon discovery, his/her corpse was subjected to a third, post-mortem examination to establish her/his "veritable" sex once and for all.

In the report of this final examination, published by Etienne Goujon in 1869, the author meticulously describes the details and ambiguities of his/her genitals, mentioning the presence of an "imperforate penis", which "in size did not exceed the clitoris of some women" (p. 134) but was nonetheless "capable of erection" (p. 131), in combination with a rudimentary vagina, ending in a cul-de-sac, in which the ejaculation of spermatozoids actually occurred. He concludes that Alexina could have played "either the masculine or the feminine role in coitus" (p. 131). The autopsy conducted on her genitals, without her consent, but described with the utmost precision, evidently raises issues of bodily integrity. Contemporary readers feel uncomfortable, as if by the act of reading they become accomplices in this post-mortem violation of a human body, committed "in the interest of science", as Goujon claims. The author almost triumphantly concludes that Alexina is "veritably" and unequivocally male, and that the autopsy has once and for all demonstrated that "hermaphroditism does not exist in man" (p. 139).[2] For Foucault (1980), this demonstrates how Victorian medicine, "with a persistence that borders on stubbornness" (1980, p. vii), tried to determine someone's "veritable sex" at all costs. Ambiguity could not be tolerated, the body had to be stripped of its "anatomical deceptions", so that science could decipher someone's

---

[2] "L'hermaphroditisme n'existe pas chez l'homme" (Goujon 1869/1978, p. 150).

true sex "hidden beneath ambiguous appearances" (p. viii). The decision to formally transfer Alexina to the "other (male) side" of society did not constitute an instance of liberation, however. Still without an unquestionable sexual identity, "he" suddenly found himself deprived of the "delights of the experience of not having one", as Foucault phrases it, of "the happy limbo of non-identity" (1980, p. xiii).

Before the rise of modern (Victorian) biomedical science, hermaphrodites had been free to decide for themselves what role they preferred to play in society or during intercourse and what sex they belonged to, Foucault argues (1980, p. vii/viii). The Victorian persistence to uphold symbolic dichotomies was complemented, however, by an obsession with genitals, for which Goujon's highly detailed account of Alexina's genitalia seems symptomatic, but this Victorian obsession is underlined by an art-work from the same era, one of the most famous artistic representations of female genitals: *L'origine du monde* ("The origin of the world"), a very detailed and realistic portrayal by Gustave Courbet (who painted it in 1866, three years before Goujon published his autopsy on Alexina Barbin) revealing a fully exposed vulva. In fact, in 1955 Jacques Lacan became the owner of Courbet's painting, who installed it in his country house in Guitrancourt, where his brother-in-law André Masson painted a board to cover it up, so that it would only be visible on special occasions (Roudinesco 1993, pp. 248–249). Notwithstanding its indisputable artistic qualities, this close-up of genitals seems an infringement of bodily integrity, much like Goujon's report. Are human genitals praised or rather desecrated by Courbet's masterpiece? Goujon's meticulously detailed description of Alexina's genitals, written in 1868, is uncannily similar to Gustave Courbet's no less detailed portrayal of the genitals of a female model (with photographic precision), dating from more or less the same period (1866). Both close-up portrayals, the artistic and the scientific one, mirror one another.

In February 2013, moreover, it was claimed, in an article in the magazine *Paris Match*, that Courbet's painting was actually a fragment, a dissected half of the original work, of which a (rediscovered) portrait of Joanna Hiffernan's (Courbet's favourite model at the time) had once formed the upper part. Courbet's portrayal of the model's face and upper body had been severed from the rest of the painting. Thus, the question emerged whether it should again be added to it, so that the art-work would be restored, that is, reunited with its purportedly missing half—a story which strangely resonates with the ancient myth told by Aristophanes at Plato's *Banquet*. Quite recently, moreover, on 25 September 2018,

Independent announced that, in a book by Claude Schopp, to be published in October 2018, it is claimed, on the basis of correspondence between Alexandre Dumas and George Sand, that the model actually was the Parisian ballet dancer Constance Queniaux. Such publications convey the desire to add a face (a) to this nameless, exposed and decapitated body, making it whole again, in accordance with Lacan's formula ($Å + a = 1$).

Aristophanes' tale and Goujon's report represent rather different types of discourse. Aristophanes relates the origins, the *genesis* of sexual identity: once upon a time, our original *nature* (φύσις) was not the same as it is now. It parodies what Lacan refers to as the *discourse of the Master*. The Master is the one who *knows*, as we have seen: a privileged, authoritative source (S_1) who knows about a mythological operation, carried out by gods. The Master knows the truth about our nature. The recipients of the message are professionals (S_2), such as a professional physician, but also a professional philosopher (Socrates), who, in Aristophanes' play *The Clouds*, is portrayed as a professional teacher in whose think-shop or thinkery (φροντιστήριο) pupils are trained in various techniques for public disputation. In short, while Aristophanes poses as Master (S_1), these professionals (the physician, the philosopher, etc.) act as the recipients of the message: $S_1 \rightarrow S_2$.

Goujon's autopsy report, however, represents a different type of discourse, referred to by Lacan as *university discourse*. Now, the professional, qualified experts themselves take the floor (S_2), and their discursive practice zooms in on a particular, partial object: Alexina's ambiguous genitals (the "object a"), reflecting the structure of university discourse ($S_2 \rightarrow a$). Rather than on the body as a whole, university discourse focuses on a very specific, partial, enigmatic, ambiguous, *impossible* object. In Courbet's painting, a particular orifice (an anonymous vulva) is regarded as a window into human "nature", into human "origins". It is an artistic enactment of the gaze of science. On closer inspection, what it brings into view is not a vulva, but rather a particular *way of seeing*, a particular gaze: the gaze of biomedical science, disclosing how human bodies were scrutinised by Victorian medicine. In Alexina's case, although his/her genitals were left intact (corrective surgery was not considered), his/her body was exposed to the gaze and instruments of modern science, via three examinations, including a post-mortem one. Once again, the focus of the expert is on a very specific, partial, enigmatic, ambiguous, impossible object: an "imperforate penis" which "in size did not exceed the clitoris of some women" but was nonetheless "capable of erection". As Lacan points out, there is an element of perversity at work in university discourse, an obsessive focus on questionable objects.

Compared to present-day biomedicine, however, the power of the Victorian gaze was limited. It was primarily descriptive and aimed at classification. Surgical interventions were not yet part of the repertoire. Victorian biomedicine lacked the capacity $(-\varphi)$ to effectively alter genitals. Goujon's aim was to align Alexina's genitals to the male-female dichotomy by *describing* them in a certain manner. Instead of a lancet, he uses his pen. This has evidently changed. Biomedicine has developed the capacity to effectively reconstruct genital organs, allegedly at will. DSD revolves around the questions whether, why and when surgical interventions are to be considered. This may even involve transplantation surgery. Just recently, in March 2018, a team of 11 surgeons at Johns Hopkins Medicine performed the world's first complete penis-and-scrotum transplant—they transplanted male genitals from a deceased donor to a recipient (an Afghanistan veteran).

My third source, again representing a different type of discourse, is the novel *Middlesex* (Eugenides 2002/2003). Here, the divided subject himself/herself is allowed to take the floor $(\$)$. The novel stages a polemic with the medical establishment, concurrent with the structure of the *discourse of the hysteric*. Calliope, a former patient, challenges biomedicine's authority to define and reconstruct gender identity. The subject takes the floor speaking in his/her own voice. The novel is a heteroglossic document, however, in the sense that various types of discourse, represented by various subjects $(\$, S_1, S_2)$ are exposed to one another. Both Aristophanes and Alexina Barbin[3] are cited and discussed, but the heart of the novel is the polemical dispute between Calliope (the divided subject, $\$$) and the psycho-medical establishment, represented by Dr Peter Luce, a prominent, professional sexologist, an *authority* in his field. What Calliope challenges, however, is not Dr Luce's expertise as such (S_2), but rather the basic views of embodiment and sexual identity which his research practice reinforces and conveys (S_1). This is how the story begins:

[3] "I may become the most famous hermaphrodite in history. Alexina Barbin, becoming Abel. Michel Foucault discovered her autobiography in the archives of the French Department of Public Hygiene. Her memoirs, which end shortly before her suicide, make unsatisfactory reading, and it was after finishing them years ago that I first got the idea to write my own" (p. 19).

Specialised readers may have come across me in Dr. Peter Luce's study, "Gender identity in 5-Alpha-Reductase Pseudo-hermaphrodites", published in the *Journal of Paediatric Endocrinology* in 1975. Or maybe you've seen my photograph in chapter sixteen of the now sadly outdated *Genetics and Heredity*. That's me on page 578, standing naked beside a height chart with a black box covering my eyes...I've been guinea-pigged by doctors, palpated by specialists... (p. 3)

From the point of view of university discourse, Calliope is a research subject in a natural experiment:

If you were going to devise an experiment to measure the relative influences of nature versus nurture, you couldn't come up with anything better than my life...Dr. Luce ran me through a barrage of tests. I was given the Benton Visual Retention Test and the Bender Visual-Motor Gestalt Test. My verbal IQ was measured. Luce even analysed my prose style to see if I wrote in a linear, masculine way, or in a circular feminine one...I am genetic history. (p. 19)

For university discourse, Calliope's genitals constitute the object *a*, the anomaly, representing questionable otherness: an anonymous, impossible object, bereft of a voice or face. In her own version of the story, Calliope parodies biomedical discourse:

By six week, I have eyes and ears. By seven, nostrils, even lips. My genitals begin to form (p. 16). Foetal hormones, taking chromosomal cues, inhibit Müllerian structures, promote Wolffian ducts. Chromosomes spinning their roulette wheels. My genes carry out their orders. All except two, a pair of miscreants—or revolutionaries—hiding out on chromosome number 5. They siphon off an enzyme, which stops the production of a certain hormone, which complicates my life. (p. 18)

The novel as such, however, focuses on his/her efforts to liberate himself/herself from this type of discourse, and from the view of embodiment and identity contained in it.

After describing his/her genitals as an anomaly (labelling his/her condition as *hypospadias*), Luce proposes to reduce the ambiguity with the help of an operation ("It was not a difficult decision, as Luce had framed it. A single surgery and some injections would give my parents back their Calliope intact", p. 429). Dr Peter Luce is an authority, as "the world's leading authority on human hermaphroditism", director of the *Sexual Disorders and Gender Identity Clinic*, which he founded in 1968, "the foremost facility in the world for the study and treatment of conditions of ambiguous gender" (p. 460). As an academic expert, Luce opts for normalisation (i.e. domestication of the *object a*), not only by re-describing Calliope's genitals, but by actively refurbishing and rearranging them ("We will finish your genitalia, they are not quite ready yet and we will finish them", p. 433). Calliope consults Webster, however, a rival source, clad in university discourse as well, and discovers an inconsistency, a crack in university discourse. In Webster it is stated that hypospadias is an abnormality of the penis, while Dr Luce insists that he/she has a clitoris. And if she had a clitoris, what could she be but a girl? Dr Luce appropriates his/her genitals by "medicalizing" them (p. 453). The inconsistency (the crack) reveals, however, that something else is at work here, guiding the discourse from beneath the bar. Again, what Calliope is contesting is not Luce's biomedical expertise as such (S_2), but rather the basic experience of embodiment, the basic body image it conveys: its guiding philosopheme (S_1 beneath the bar). Dr Luce's theory of gender identity reflects the ideology of the early seventies, when the consensus was that identity is primarily determined by environment, and each child was considered a blank slate (p. 478):

> Women were becoming more like men and men were becoming more like women. For a little while it seemed that sexual difference might pass away. But then another thing happened. It was called evolutionary biology. Under its sway, the sexes were separated again, men into hunters and women into gatherers. Nurture no longer formed us, nature did. Impulses from hominids dating from 20,000 B.C. were still controlling us. Men and women wanted to be different again. Dr. Luce's theory had come under attack by the 1990s. Every newborn had been inscribed by genetics and evolution. My life exists at the center of this debate. (p. 479)

During the 1970s, environment (nurture) was seen as the determining factor, but during the 1990s (the era of the *Human Genome Project*), genetical determinism was in sway, reflecting a shift beneath the bar, affecting the basic orientation, university discourse's guiding philosopheme, from *nurture* to *nature*. But then there was another dialectical pendulum swing (Nelkin and Lindee 1995/2004; Zwart 2007, 2014): "[C]ontrary to all expectations, the code underlying our being failed to live up to expectations. Instead of the expected 200,000 genes, humans have only 30,000" (p. 479). And so, a strange new possibility was arising:

free will made a comeback—"biology gives you a brain, life turns it into a mind" (p. 479). Sexuality became a practice of the Self again ("I began experimenting with myself", p. 453).

To escape the reign of university discourse and its interpretation of embodiment, Calliope leaves home and hits the road to California, towards self-discovery (to discover who she is and what she really wants). She enters the porno scene, exposing himself/herself as an anomaly inside a tank filled with water, but viewers never see the whole body, only partial objects, "only pieces...a knee, for example, or a nipple" (p. 480). And even if they see "the source of life, the thing of things", they see it "purified as it were, without the clutter of a person attached" (p. 480). For Calliope, this is a practice of the Self: it is "therapeutic" (p. 494). In Foucauldian terms, it is *ars erotica*, an exercise to escape Dr Luce's *scientia sexualis* (Foucault 1976). At first, Dr Luce is desperate, as if he has lost his greatest find. Later he realises that Calliope does not support his theories at all (p. 479). And now he hopes she will stay quiet and never show up as a living refutation of his papers (p. 479).

In Lacanian terms, the novel reflects a shift from *university discourse* (bent on domesticating the anomalous object *a*), via the *discourse of the hysteric* (involving a desperate, divided subject who challenges the basic convictions of the biomedical establishment) towards the *discourse of the analyst* (a process of auto-analysis and working through). In the discourse of the analyst, biomedical expertise (the biomedical gaze: S_2) is silenced/bracketed (pushed beneath the bar), so that the object *a* comes into view as the thing which sets his/her life in motion. Calliope's life revolves around an enigmatic erogenous object, an anomaly, which tends to be hidden, but attracts Dr Luce's attention (*a*), while also constituting a challenge for Calliope himself/herself as a divided subject ($\$$), involving him/her in a process of individuation, portrayed minutiously in the course of the novel (Fig. 22.1).

From the point of view of the discourse of the analyst, the narrative revolves around the object *a*, assuming a semblance of agency, something Calliope has to come to terms with. To achieve this, biomedical and sexology expertise must be suspended (S_2 pushed into the lower-left position), while the by-product of the process is a new understanding of embodiment which challenges the biomedical view of the re-makeable body (S_1). Thus, the basic structure of the novel can be presented as shown in Fig. 22.2.

Fig. 22.1 *Middlesex*: The discourse of the analyst

a	$\$$
S_2	S_1

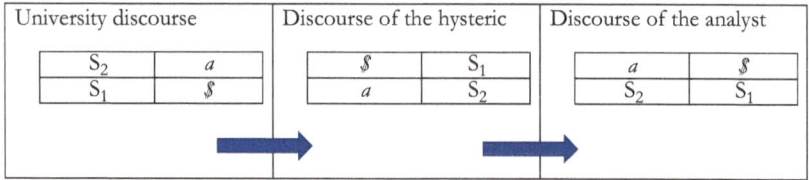

University discourse		Discourse of the hysteric		Discourse of the analyst	
S_2	a	$\$$	S_1	a	$\$$
S_1	$\$$	a	S_2	S_2	S_1

Fig. 22.2 *Middlesex*: Basic structure

The novel sets off as a critical exposition of a particular scientific research practice (sexology) as it appeared on the scene during the 1970s: a particular configuration of knowledge, represented by Dr Luce as agent/expert (S_2), addressing a particular partial object (a), Calliope's genitals. It is a *critical* exposition, however, revealing the basic conviction, the *philosopheme* (S_1) at work in this discourse, while also fleshing out the physical and mental discontent ($\$$) it produces. This discourse is subverted, however, when Calliope (the divided subject) takes the floor to challenge Luce's understanding of embodiment and identity, not only verbally, but also via a *passage à l'acte*, a practice of the Self, a series of therapeutic exercises (Go West!), an auto-analysis if you like, concurrent with the discourse of the analyst: bracketing academic expertise (S_2) and focusing on the interaction between the object (the object a, the partial organ) and the divided subject, contributing to the dawning of a new vision of embodiment (S_1).

REFERENCES

Beh, H.G., and M. Diamond. 2000. An Emerging Ethical and Medical Dilemma: Should Physicians Perform Sex Assignment Surgery on Infants with Ambiguous Genitalia? *Michigan Journal of Gender and Law* 7 (1): 1–63.

Domurat Dreger, A. 1998. Ambiguous Sex – or Ambivalent Medicine? *The Hastings Center Report* 28 (3): 24–35.

Eugenides, J. 2002/2003. *Middlesex*. London: Bloomsbury.

Foucault, M. 1976. *Histoire de la sexualité I: La volonté de savoir*. Paris: Gallimard.

———. 1978. *Herculine Barbin dite Alexina B.* Paris: Gallimard.

———. 1980. Introduction. In *Herculine Barbin, Being the Recently Rediscovered Memoirs of a Nineteenth-Century French Hermaphrodite*, ed. Michel Foucault, vii–xvii. New York: Pantheon Books.

Freud, S. 1920/1940. Jenseits des Lustprinzips. In *Gesammelte Werke XIII*, 1–70. London: Imago.

Goujon, E. 1869/1978. Étude d'un cas d'hermaphroditisme imparfait chez l'homme. In *Herculine Barbin dite Alexina B*, ed. M. Foucault, 141–154. Paris: Gallimard.

Kipnis, K., and M. Diamond. 1998. Pediatric Ethics and the Surgical Assignment of Sex. *Journal of Clinical Ethics* 9: 398–410.

Lacan, J. 1966. *Écrits*. Paris: Éditions du Seuil.

Lee, P.A., C.P. Houk, S.F. Ahmed, and I.A. Hughes. 2006. Consensus Statement on Management of Intersex Disorders. *Pediatrics* 118: e488–e500. https://doi.org/10.1542/peds.2006-0738.

Masson, J. 1984/2003. *The Assault on Truth: Freud's Suppression of the Seduction Theory*. New York: Ballantine Books.

Nelkin, D., and S. Lindee. 1995/2004. *The DNA Mystique: The Gene as a Cultural Icon*. Ann Arbor: University of Michigan Press.

Reik, T. 1960. *The Creation of Woman: A Psychoanalytic Inquiry into the Myth of Eve*. New York: McGraw-Hill.

Roudinesco, E. 1993. *Jacques Lacan: Esquisse d'une vie, histoire d'un système de pensée*. Paris: Fayard.

Tardieu, A. 1872. *Question médico-légale de l'identité dans ses rapports avec les vices de conformation des organes sexuels, contenant les souvenirs et impressions d'un individu dont le sexe avait été méconnu*, 48–159. Paris: Ballière.

Wiesemann, C., S. Ude-Koeller, G. Sinnecker, and U. Thyen. 2010. Ethical Principles and Recommendations for the Medical Management of Differences of Sex Development (DSD)/Intersex in Children and Adolescents. *European Journal of Pediatrics* 169: 671–679.

Zwart, H. 2007. Genomics and Self-Knowledge: Implications for Societal Research and Debate. *New Genetics and Society* 26 (2): 181–202.

———. 2014. Book Review: The DNA Mystique: The Gene as a Cultural Icon. *Sociology* 47 (5): 1030–1032.

REFERENCES

Adler, A. 1917/1927. *Studie über Minderwertigkeit von Organen.* Darmstadt: Wissenschaftliche Buchgesellschaft.

———. 1927/2009. *Menschenkenntnis.* Frankfurt am Main: Fischer.

Althusser, L., and E. Balibar. 1970. *Lire le capital.* Paris: Maspero.

Appadurai, A. 1986. *The Social Life of Things.* New York: Cambridge University Press.

Aquinas, T. 1922. *Summa Theologica.* Taurini: Marietti.

Awaya, T. 1994. The Theory of Neo-Cannibalism. *Japanese Journal of Philosophy* 3: 29–47.

Beh, H.G., and M. Diamond. 2000. An Emerging Ethical and Medical Dilemma: Should Physicians Perform Sex Assignment Surgery on Infants with Ambiguous Genitalia? *Michigan Journal of Gender and Law* 7 (1): 1–63.

van den Berg, J.H. 1961. *Het menselijk lichaam: een metabletisch onderzoek 2: Het verlaten lichaam.* Nijkerk: Callenbach.

Beugnet, M. 2008. The Practice of Strangeness: L'Intrus – Claire Denis (2004) and Jean-Luc Nancy (2000). *Film-Philosophy* 12 (1): 31–48.

Blackman, L. 2010. Bodily Integrity. *Body & Society* 16 (3): 1–9.

Bogdanov, A. 1908/1984. *Red Star.* Bloomington: University of Indiana Press.

Bracher, M., M. Alcorn, F. Massardier-Kennedy, and R. Corthell, eds. 1994. *Lacanian Theory of Discourse: Subject, Structure, and Society.* New York: New York University Press.

Burnet, F.M. 1963. *The Integrity of the Body.* Cambridge: Harvard University Press.

Carney, S. 2011. *The Red Market: On the Trail of the World's Organ Brokers, Bone Thieves, Blood Farmers, and Child Traffickers.* New York: HarperCollins.

© The Author(s) 2019

H. A. E. Zwart, *Purloined Organs,*

https://doi.org/10.1007/978-3-030-05354-3

Cassell, E. 1992. The Body of the Future. In *The Body in Medical Thought and Practice*, Philosophy & Medicine, ed. D. Leder, vol. 43, 233–249. Dordrecht/Boston/London: Kluwer.

Coeckelbergh, M. 2015. The Art of Living with ICTs: The Ethics–Aesthetics of Vulnerability Coping and Its Implications for Understanding and Evaluating ICT Cultures. *Foundations of Science* 22 (2): 339–348.

Cook, R. 1977. *Coma*. New York: Little, Brown & Co.

Dautzenberg, A.H.J. 2011. *Samaritaan*. Amsterdam/Antwerp: Contact.

Declaration of Istanbul on Organ Trafficking and Transplant Tourism. 2008. *Kidney International* 74 (7): 854–859.

Dekkers, W., and H. ten Have. 1998. Biomedical Research with Human Body 'Parts'. In *Ownership of the Human Body: Philosophical Considerations of the Human Body and Its Parts in Healthcare*, ed. H. ten Have and J. Welie, 49–63. Dordrecht/Boston/London: Kluwer.

Den Hartogh, G. 2013a. Is Consent of the Donor Enough to Justify the Removal of Living Organs? *Cambridge Quarterly of Healthcare Ethics* 22 (1): 45–54.

———. 2013b. The Political Obligation to Donate Organs. *Ratio Juris* 26 (3): 378–403.

Diderot, D. 1769/1951. *Le rêve de d'Alembert: entretien entre d'Alembert et Diderot*. Société des textes français modernes. Paris: Didier.

Dixon, L. 1981. Bosch's Garden of Delights Triptych: Remnants of a Fossil Science. *The Art Bulletin* 63 (1): 96–113.

Domurat Dreger, A. 1998. Ambiguous Sex – or Ambivalent Medicine? *The Hastings Center Report* 28 (3): 24–35.

Erin, C., and J. Harris. 2003. An Ethical Market in Human Organs. *Journal of Medical Ethics* 29: 137–138.

Eugenides, J. 2002/2003. *Middlesex*. London: Bloomsbury.

Foucault, M. 1976. *Histoire de la sexualité I: La volonté de savoir*. Paris: Gallimard.

———. 1978. *Herculine Barbin dite Alexina B*. Paris: Gallimard.

———. 1980. Introduction. In *Herculine Barbin, Being the Recently Rediscovered Memoirs of a Nineteenth-Century French Hermaphrodite*, ed. Michel Foucault, vii–xvii. New York: Pantheon Books.

———. 1994. A propos de la généalogie de l'éthique. In *Dits et Écrits IV*, 383–411. Paris: Gallimard.

Frazer, J. 1890/1993. *The Golden Bough*. London: Wordsworth.

Freud, S. 1895/1952. Studien über Hysterie. In *Gesammelte Werke I*, 75–312. London: Imago.

———. 1900/1942. Die Traumdeutung. In *Gesammelte Werke II/III*. London: Imago.

———. 1905/1942. Drei Abhandlungen zur Sexualtheorie. In *Gesammelte Werke V*, 27–145. London: Imago.

———. 1907/1941. Der Wahn und die Träume in W. Jensens *Gradiva*. In *Gesammelte Werke VII*, 29–122. London: Imago.

———. 1913/1940. Totem und Tabu. In *Gesammelte Werke IX*. London: Imago.

———. 1919/1947. Das Unheimliche. In *Gesammelte Werke XII*, 227–268. London: Imago.

———. 1920/1940. Jenseits des Lustprinzips. In *Gesammelte Werke XIII*, 1–70. London: Imago.

———. 1921/1940. Massenpsychologie und Ich-Analyse. In *Gesammelte Werke XIII*, 71–162. London: Imago.

———. 1923/1940. Das Ich und das Es. In *Gesammelte Werke XIII*, 237–289. London: Imago.

———. 1930/1948. Das Unbehagen in der Kultur. In *Gesammelte Werke XIV*, 419–513. London: Imago.

Gehlen, A. 1940/1962. *Der Mensch. Seine Natur und seine Stellung in der Welt*. Frankfurt: Athenäum.

Goujon, E. 1869/1978. Étude d'un cas d'hermaphroditisme imparfait chez l'homme. In *Herculine Barbin dite Alexina B*, ed. M. Foucault, 141–154. Paris: Gallimard.

Grant, E. 1974. *A Source Book in Medieval Science*. Harvard: Harvard University Press.

Greenberg, O. 2013. The Global Organ Trade. *Cambridge Quarterly of Healthcare Ethics* 22 (3): 238–245.

Groys, B., and M. Hagemeister. 2005. *Die neue Menschheit: Biopolitische Utopien in Russland zu Beginn des 20*. Jahrhunderts. Frankfurt am Main: Suhrkamp.

Gunkel, D., and P. Taylor. 2014. *Heidegger and the Media*. Cambridge: Polity.

Hagen, P.J. 1982. *Blood: Gift or Merchandise; Towards an International Blood Policy*. New York: Liss.

Horbach, S., and W. Halffman. 2017. The Ghosts of HeLa: How Cell Line Misidentification Contaminates the Scientific Literature. *PLoS One* 12 (10): e0186281. https://doi.org/10.1371/journal.pone.0186281.

Hurst, S. 2015. The Ethics of Selling Body Parts. In *New Cannibal Markets: Globalization and Commodification of the Human Body*, ed. J.-D. Rainhorn and S. Boudamoussi, 47–56. Paris: Maison des sciences de l'homme.

Kant, I. 1785/1980. Grundlegung zur Metaphysik der Sitten. In *Werkausgabe 7*. Frankfurt am Main: Suhrkamp.

Kass, L. 1992. Organs for Sale? Propriety, Property, and the Price of Progress. *The Public Interest* Spring (107): 65–86.

Kipnis, K., and M. Diamond. 1998. Pediatric Ethics and the Surgical Assignment of Sex. *Journal of Clinical Ethics* 9: 398–410.

de Kruif, P. 1945/1948. *The Male Hormone*. New York: Permabooks/Harcourt & Brace.

Lacan, J. 1938/2001. Les complexes familiaux dans la formation de l'individu: Essai d'analyse d'une fonction en psychologie. In *Autres Écrits*, 23–84. Paris: Éditions du Seuil.

———. 1955–1956/1981. *Le Séminaire de Jacques Lacan III: Les psychoses*. Paris: Éditions du Seuil.

————. 1956–1957/1994. *Le Séminaire de Jacques Lacan IV: La relation d'objet et les structures freudiennes.* Paris: Éditions du Seuil.

————. 1959–1960/1986. *Le Séminaire de Jacques Lacan VII: L'éthique de la psychanalyse.* Paris: Éditions du Seuil.

————. 1962–1963/2004. *Le Séminaire de Jacques Lacan X: L'Angoisse.* Paris: Éditions du Seuil.

————. 1964/1973. *Le séminaire de Jacques Lacan XI: Les quatre concepts fondamentaux de la psychanalyse.* Paris: Éditions du Seuil.

————. 1966a. *Écrits.* Paris: Éditions du Seuil.

————. 1966b. Kant avec Sade. In *Écrits*, 765–790. Paris: Éditions du Seuil.

————. 1966–1967. *Le séminaire XIV: Logique du fantasme* (unpublished). http://staferla.free.fr/.

————. 1967–1968. *Le Séminaire de Jacques Lacan XV: L'acte de la psychanalyse* (unpublished). http://staferla.free.fr/.

————. 1968–1969/2006. *Le Séminaire de Jacques Lacan XVI: D'un Autre à l'autre.* Paris: Éditions du Seuil.

————. 1969–1970/1991. *Le séminaire XVII: L'envers de la psychanalyse.* Paris: Éditions du Seuil.

————. 1971–1972. *Le savoir du psychoanalyst* (unpublished seminar). http://www.valas.fr/.

Lane, N. 2005. *Power, Sex, Suicide: Mitochondria and the Meaning of Life.* Oxford/New York: Oxford University Press.

Lee, P.A., C.P. Houk, S.F. Ahmed, and I.A. Hughes. 2006. Consensus Statement on Management of Intersex Disorders. *Pediatrics* 118: e488–e500. https://doi.org/10.1542/peds.2006-0738.

Lemmens, P. 2015. Social Autonomy and Heteronomy in the Age of ICT: The Digital Pharmakon and the (Dis)Empowerment of the General Intellect. *Foundations of Science* 22 (2): 287–296. https://doi.org/10.1007/s10699-015-9468-1.

Livingston, P. 2006. Theses on Cinema as Philosophy. *The Journal of Aesthetics and Art Criticism* 64 (1): 11–18.

Lock, M. 2002. *Twice Dead: Organ Transplants and the Reinvention of Death.* Berkeley/Los Angeles/California: University of California Press.

Marx, K. 1867/1979. *Das Kapital. Kritik der politischen Oekonomie 1: der produktionsprocess des Kapitals.* Berlin: Dietz.

Masson, J. 1984/2003. *The Assault on Truth: Freud's Suppression of the Seduction Theory.* New York: Ballantine Books.

Matas, D., and T. Trey. 2012. *Transplant Abuse in China.* Niagara Falls: Seraphim Editions.

Merleau-Ponty, M. 1945. *Phénoménologie de la perception.* Paris: Gallimard.

Meyer, S. 2006. Trafficking in Human Organs in Europe: A Myth or an Actual Threat? *European Journal of Crime, Criminal Law & Criminal Justice* 14 (2): 208–229.

Miller, J.-A. 2001. Lacanian Biology and the Event of the Body. *Lacanian Ink* 18: 6–29.

Morrey, D. 2008a. Introduction: Claire Denis and Jean-Luc Nancy. *Film-Philosophy* 12 (1): i–vi.

———. 2008b. Open Wounds: Body and Image in Jean-Luc Nancy and Claire Denis. *Film-Philosophy* 12 (1): 10–31.

Nancy, J.-L. 2000/2010. *L'intrus*. Paris: Galilée.

———. 2005. *L'Intrus selon Claire Denis*. Remue.net: http://remue.net/spip.php?article679.

Nelkin, D., and S. Lindee. 1995/2004. *The DNA Mystique: The Gene as a Cultural Icon*. Ann Arbor: University of Michigan Press.

Plato. 1925/1996. *Lysis, Symposium, Gorgias*. Loeb ed. Cambridge: Harvard University Press.

Rabinow, P. 1996. *Essays on the Anthropology of Reason*. Princeton: Princeton University Press.

Ragland, E. 1995. The Relation Between the Voice and the Gaze. In *Reading Seminar XI: Lacan's Four Fundamental Concepts of Psychoanalysis*, ed. Richard Feldstein, Bruce Fink, and Maire Jaanus, 187–203. Albany: State University of New York Press.

Reik, T. 1960. *The Creation of Woman: A Psychoanalytic Inquiry into the Myth of Eve*. New York: McGraw-Hill.

Rheeder, R. 2017. A Global Bioethical Perspective on Organ Trafficking: Discrimination, Stigmatisation and the Vulnerable. *South Africa Journal of Bioethics and Law* 10 (1): 20–24. https://doi.org/10.7196/SAJBL.2017.v10i1.528.

Richardson, R. 1996. Fearful Symmetry: Corpses for Anatomy, Organs for Transplantation? In *Organ Transplantation: Meanings and Realities*, ed. S. Youngner, R. Fox, and L. O'Connell, 66–100. Madison: University of Wisconsin Press.

Roudinesco, E. 1993. *Jacques Lacan: Esquisse d'une vie, histoire d'un système de pensée*. Paris: Fayard.

Scheper-Hughes, N. 2000. The Global Traffic in Human Organs. *Current Anthropology* 41: 191–224.

———. 2002. The Ends of the Body: Commodity Fetishism and the Global Traffic in Organs. *SAIS Review* 22 (1): 61–80.

———. 2008. *The Last Commodity: Post-Human Ethics, Global (In)Justice and the Traffic in Organs*. Penang: Multiversity & Citizens International.

Schicktanz, S., C. Wiesemann, and S. Wöhlke. 2010. *Teaching Ethics in Organ Transplantation and Tissue Donation Cases and Movies*. Göttingen: Universitätsverlag.

Schweda, M., and S. Schicktanz. 2009. The 'Spare Parts Person'? Conceptions of the Human Body and Their Implications for Public Attitudes Towards

Organ Donation and Organ Sale. *Philosophy, Ethics, and Humanities in Medicine* 4 (4): 1–10.

Sharif, A., M. Fiatarone Singh, T. Trey, and J. Lavee. 2014. Organ Procurement from Executed Prisoners in China. *American Journal of Transplantation* 14: 2246–2252.

Sharp, L. 2006. *Strange Harvest: Organ Transplants, Denatured Bodies and the Transformed Self*. Berkeley/Los Angeles/London: University of California Press.

———. 2007. *Bodies, Commodities and Biotechnologies. Death, Mourning and Scientific Desire in the Realm of Human Organ Transfer*. New York: Columbia University Press.

Shildrick, M. 2010. Some Reflections on the Socio-Cultural and Bioscientific Limits of Bodily Integrity. *Body & Society* 16 (3): 11–22.

Shimazono, Y. 2007. The State of the International Organ Trade: A Provisional Picture Based on Integration of Available Information. *Bulletin of the WHO* 85 (12). https://doi.org/10.1590/S0042-96862007001200017.

Skloot, R. 2011. *The Immortal Life of Henrietta Lacks*. New York: Broadway Paperbacks.

Slatman, J., and G. Widdershoven. 2010. Hand Transplants and Bodily Integrity. *Body & Society* 16 (3): 69–92.

Sloterdijk, P. 1998. *Sphären I: Blasen*. Frankfurt: Suhrkamp.

———. 2009. *Du musst dein Leben ändern: Über Anthropotechnik*. Frankfurt: Suhrkamp.

Sloterdijk, P., and H.-J. Heinrichs. 2001. *Die Sonne und der Tod: Dialogische Untersuchungen*. Frankfurt: Suhrkamp.

Starzl, T. 1992/2003. *The Puzzle People. Memoirs of a Transplant Surgeon*. Pittsburgh/London: University of Pittsburgh Press.

Stenner, P., and E. Moreno-Gabriel. 2013. Liminality and Affectivity: The Case of Deceased Organ Donation. *Subjectivity* 6 (3): 229–253.

Stiegler, B. 2010. *Ce qui fait que la vie vaut la peine d'être vécue: de la pharmacologie*. Paris: Flammarion.

Stoker, B. 1897/1993. *Dracula*. Hertfordshire: Wordsworth.

Streiter, A. 2008. The Community According to Jean-Luc Nancy and Claire Denis. *Film-Philosophy* 12 (1): 49–62.

Sweeney, R.E. 2005. The Hither Side of Solutions: Bodies and Landscape in *L'Intrus*. *Senses of Cinema* 36. http://sensesofcinema.com/2005/feature-articles/intrus/.

Tardieu, A. 1872. *Question médico-légale de l'identité dans ses rapports avec les vices de conformation des organes sexuels, contenant les souvenirs et impressions d'un individu dont le sexe avait été méconnu*, 48–159. Paris: Ballière.

Ten Have, H., and J. Welie. 1998. *Ownership of the Human Body: Philosophical Considerations of the Human Body and Its Parts in Healthcare*. Dordrecht/Boston/London: Kluwer.

Titmuss, R.M. 1971. *The Gift Relationship: From Human Blood to Social Policy.* London: Allen & Unwin.

Van Assche, K. 2018. Combating the Trade in Organs: Why Should We Preserve the Communal Nature of Organ Transplantation. In *Personalized Medicine, Individual Choice and the Common Good,* ed. B. van Beers, D. Dickenson, and S. Sterckx, 77–112. Cambridge: Cambridge University Press.

Varela, F. 2001. Intimate Distances: Fragments for a Phenomenology of Organ Transplantation. *Journal of Consciousness Studies* 8 (5–7): 259–271.

Verhaeghe, P. 2001. *Beyond Gender: From Subject to Drive.* New York: Other Press.

Waldby, C. 2002. Biomedicine, Tissue Transfer and Intercorporeality. *Feminist Theory* 3: 235–250.

Waldby, C., and R. Mitchell. 2006. *Tissue Economies: Blood, Organs and Cell Lines in Late Capitalism.* Durham & London: Duke University Press.

Wiesemann, C., S. Ude-Koeller, G. Sinnecker, and U. Thyen. 2010. Ethical Principles and Recommendations for the Medical Management of Differences of Sex Development (DSD)/Intersex in Children and Adolescents. *European Journal of Pediatrics* 169: 671–679.

Wollstonecraft Shelley, M. 1818/1968. *Frankenstein; or, the Modern Prometheus.* Harmondsworth: Penguin.

Yoshizawa, K., R. Ferreira, Y. Kamimura, and C. Lienhard. 2014. Female Penis, Male Vagina, and Their Correlated Evolution in a Cave Insect. *Current Biology* 24: 1–5. https://doi.org/10.1016/j.cub.2014.03.022.

Young, I.M. 1992. Breasted Experience: The Look and the Feeling. In *The Body in Medical Thought and Practice,* Philosophy & Medicine, ed. Drew Leder, vol. 43, 215–230. Dordrecht/Boston/London: Kluwer.

Žižek, S. 2004/2012. *Organs Without Bodies: On Deleuze and Consequences.* London/New York: Routledge.

———. 2006/2009. *The Parallax View.* Cambridge/London: The MIT Press

———. 2010. *Living in the End Times.* London/New York: Verso.

Zwart, H. 1997. What Is an Animal? A Philosophical Reflection on the Possibility of a Moral Relationship with Animals. *Environmental Values* 6 (4): 377–392.

———. 1998. Medicine, Symbolization and the 'Real Body': Lacan's Understanding of Medical Science. *Medicine, Healthcare and Philosophy: A European Journal* 1 (2): 107–117.

———. 2000. From Circle to Square: Integrity, Vulnerability and Digitalization. In *Bioethics and Law II: Four Ethical Principles,* ed. P. Kemp et al., 141–153. Copenhagen: Rhodos.

———. 2002. *Boude bewoordingen. De historische fenomenologie van J.H. van den Berg.* Kampen: Klement/Kapellen: Pelckmans. ISBN 90 77070 26 5.

———. 2007. Genomics and Self-Knowledge: Implications for Societal Research and Debate. *New Genetics and Society* 26 (2): 181–202.

———. 2009. From Utopia to Science: Challenges of Personalised Genomics Information for Health Management and Health Enhancement. *Medicine Studies* 1 (2): 155–166.

———. 2012. On Decoding and Rewriting Genomes: A Psychoanalytical Reading of a Scientific Revolution. *Medicine, Healthcare and Philosophy: A European Journal* 15 (3): 337–346.

———. 2014a. The Donor Organ as an 'Object A': A Lacanian Perspective on Organ Donation and Transplantation Medicine. *Medicine, Health Care & Philosophy: A European Journal* 17 (4): 559–571. https://doi.org/10.1007/s11019-014-9553-1.

———. 2014b. Book Review: The DNA Mystique: The Gene as a Cultural Icon. *Sociology* 47 (5): 1030–1032.

———. 2015. A New Lease on Life: A Lacanian Analysis of Cognitive Enhancement Cinema. In *Handbook Posthumanism in Film and Television*, ed. Michael Hauskeller et al., 214–224. London: Palgrave Macmillan.

———. 2016a. Transplantation Medicine, Organ Theft Cinema and Bodily Integrity. *Subjectivity* 9 (2): 151–180. https://doi.org/10.1057/sub.2016.1.

———. 2016b. The Obliteration of Life: Depersonalisation and Disembodiment in the Terabyte Age. *New Genetics and Society* 35 (1): 69–89. https://doi.org/10.1080/14636778.2016.1143770.

———. 2016c. Psychoanalysis and Bioethics: A Lacanian Approach to Bioethical Discourse. *Medicine, Healthcare and Philosophy* 19 (4): 605–621. https://doi.org/10.1007/s11019-016-9698-1.

———. 2017a. The Oblique Perspective: Philosophical Diagnostics of Contemporary Life Sciences Research. *Life Sciences, Society & Policy* 13 (1): 1–20. https://doi.org/10.1186/s40504-017-0047-9.

———. 2017b. Extimate' Technologies and Techno-Cultural Discontent: A Lacanian Analysis of Pervasive Gadgets. *Techné: Research in Philosophy and Technology* 21 (1): 24–54. https://doi.org/10.5840/techne2017456.

———. 2017c. *Tales of Research Misconduct: A Lacanian Diagnostics of Integrity Challenges in Science Novels.* Library of Ethics and Applied Philosophy. Cham: Springer. https://doi.org/10.1007/978-3-319-65554-3

———. 2018. Vampires, Viruses and Verbalisation: Bram Stoker's Dracula as a Genealogical Window into Fin-De-Siècle Science. *Janus Head: Journal of Interdisciplinary Studies in Literature, Continental Philosophy, Phenomenological Psychology, and the Arts* 16 (2): 14–53.

Zwart, H., and C. Hoffer. 1998. *Orgaandonatie en lichamelijke integriteit.* Best: Damon.

Index[1]

---

[1] Note: Page numbers followed by 'n' refer to notes.

© The Author(s) 2019   137
H. A. E. Zwart, *Purloined Organs*,
https://doi.org/10.1007/978-3-030-05354-3